Suicide-Related Behaviour

Copyright © 2007   John Wiley & Sons Ltd,
                      The Atrium, Southern Gate, Chichester,
                      West Sussex PO19 8SQ, England

                      Telephone   (+44) 1243 779777

Email (for orders and customer service enquiries): cs-books@wiley.co.uk
Visit our Home Page on www.wiley.com

Other Wiley Editorial Offices

John Wiley & Sons Inc., 111 River Street, Hoboken, NJ 07030, USA

Jossey-Bass, 989 Market Street, San Francisco, CA 94103-1741, USA

Wiley-VCH Verlag GmbH, Boschstr. 12, D-69469 Weinheim, Germany

John Wiley & Sons Australia Ltd, 42 McDougall Street, Milton, Queensland 4064, Australia

John Wiley & Sons (Asia) Pte Ltd, 2 Clementi Loop #02-01, Jin Xing Distripark, Singapore 129809

John Wiley & Sons Canada Ltd, 6045 Freemont Blvd, Mississauga, ONT, L5R 4J3, Canada

Wiley also publishes its books in a variety of electronic formats. Some content that appears in print may not be available in electronic books.

Anniversary Logo Design: Richard J. Pacifico

Library of Congress Cataloging-in-Publication Data

McLaughlin, Columba.
    Suicide-related behaviours: understanding, caring, and therapeutic responses / Columba McLaughlin.
        p. ; cm.
    Includes bibliographical references and index.
    ISBN 978-1-86156-508-2 (pbk. : alk. paper)
    1. Suicidal behavior. 2. Suicidal behavior–Psychological aspects. 3. Suicidal behavior–Treatment.
I. Title.
    [DNLM: 1. Suicide, Attempted–psychology. 2. Adolescent. 3. Self-Injurious Behavior–therapy.
WM 165 M478s 2007]
    RC569.M42 2007
    616.85'8445–dc22

                                                                2007006009

British Library Cataloguing in Publication Data

A catalogue record for this book is available from the British Library

ISBN 978-1-86156-508-2

Typeset in 9.5/13pt Photina MT by SNP Best-set Typesetter Ltd., Hong Kong
Printed and bound in Great Britain by TJ International Ltd, Padstow, Cornwall

This book is printed on acid-free paper responsibly manufactured from sustainable forestry in which at least two trees are planted for each one used for paper production.

Suicide-Related Behaviour – Understanding, Caring and Therapeutic Responses

COLUMBA McLAUGHLIN

John Wiley & Sons, Ltd

Dedication

This book is dedicated to those friends whom I was very fortunate to meet before they decided to leave

Acknowledgements

For my parents John and Millie who were always there for me. Also for the patience of my wife Deirdre and my children who encouraged me to write this book. In addition, I would like to acknowledge my thanks to Professor Dorothy Whittington for her supervision, Professor Hugh McKenna and Professor Kader Parahoo for their encouragement, the library staff in the University of Ulster and the staff in the Barnes Unit for their mentorship and help in my understanding of this emotional and very human subject. In particular the following: Karen, Dave, Jill, Margaret and especially Professor Keith Hawton who all gave me the opportunity to learn in the early days of suicidology. You will not be forgotten.

Useful notes when using this book

1. In this book the term 'person' will frequently be used to refer to someone who is in psychological distress and has sought help from statutory or voluntary health care services. The term 'client' is used when necessary and when referring specifically to persons who are in therapy. This is done to prevent changing between numerous other terms such as consumer, client, patient, service user, or expert by experience.

2. Also, most of the case studies in this book are based on real people and on real events. In all case studies in this book, pseudonyms are used and some personal details are changed in order to provide anonymity.

3. The term 'practitioner' will be used to refer to all those people who provide mental health care to persons in psychological distress, such as nurses, social workers, psychologists, psychiatrists, therapists, occupational therapists, counsellors/psychotherapists or other support workers. Occupational titles will only be used when referring to research articles that involve specific professions.

4. Parts of this book deal with the therapeutic relationship between the client and the practitioner. Also, the book introduces the reader to communication skills and to some basic counselling/psychotherapy techniques. It is emphasized here that the basic knowledge in this book is not a substitute for such specialized knowledge or courses. Readers who have an interest in counselling/psychotherapy should seek additional training and supervised practice in these highly specialized courses.

Contents

Preface

This book has been, for me, a long time in the writing. The phenomenon of suicide-related behaviour has fascinated me since my late teens and I have for a long time striven to understand issues within it. In a way, this book is an attempt to make sense of suicide-related behaviour in terms of understanding its aetiology and how practitioners can respond in a caring and therapeutic manner. I have written this book for those students who are considering a career in mental health care. Such students, to name but a few, would include nurses, medical students, social workers, psychologists, occupational therapists and other related mental health practitioners. In this book the term practitioner will refer to all those professionals, both qualified and students, who are involved in the physical and psychological care of people who self-harm or attempt suicide. Just like other professionals currently involved in mental health, they are now beginning their journey into mental health care and mental health promotion.

Without doubt, there is no greater problem facing mental health practitioners than suicide-related behaviour. Over the last thirty years the data gathered have consistently indicated that suicide is a leading cause of death in our young people. This is especially so of young men. Currently, the data indicate that in some areas suicide is increasing. Alongside this, the incidence of self-harm, which has always been high, does not seem to be abating. Some professionals argue that attempted suicide and self-harm are both the same entity. In this book, it is put forward that they are two sides of the same coin and this coin is called suicide-related behaviour. In effect, the term suicide-related behaviour is a general term used in this book to describe all behaviours where the person intended to kill or harm him/her self. In so doing, relevant issues within the phenomenon of suicide-related behaviour, and specific to both self-harm and attempted suicide, will be explored and addressed in this book.

In Chapter 1 of this book and in an effort to show the varying differences within the concept of suicide-related behaviour, I have reflected on some of my experiences of people who allowed me to share their lives. In Chapter 2, it is well recognized that the phenomenon of suicide-related behaviour is a very controversial subject and is frequently seen as a contradiction in terms. As well, in recent times the concept of euthanasia and physician-assisted suicide have come to the fore. Another difficult issue is that of attitudes to suicide-related behaviour. In Chapter 2, these contemporary issues are explored through discussion and through student exercises. In Chapter 3, there is within the phenomenon of suicide-related behaviour a varying number of terms used to describe the methods that people employ to kill themselves, attempt suicide or self-harm. Many of these terms have been brought about with good intention by well-meaning authors. However, occasionally the interpretation of these terms can create thorny definitional discussions between practitioners from different health care professions. An exploration of the terms used is carried out in Chapter 3. In addition, Chapter 3 introduces the reader to the concept of suicide-related behaviour.

In Chapter 4, the term suicide-related behaviour and what it means is reflected on, described and discussed. Examples are used to enhance understanding. Following this, in Chapter 5, how a person can arrive on the brink of crisis and consider suicide-related behaviour as an option is discussed. This chapter explores the person's descent into crisis from a number of different perspectives. Chapter 6 looks at some of the person's responses to crisis. These responses range from the biological, psychological and the social. It also explores different buffers that protect the human psyche from the worst ravages of life events. In Chapter 7, the case for a caring response and the qualities needed in practitioners are explored. Also, the skills required are outlined and an example of a caring/therapeutic response is given. In Chapter 8, the medical response is discussed and an argument is put for an in-depth assessment. In addition, an example of a therapeutic model is applied and there is also a brief introduction to merits of cognitive behavioural therapy. Finally, Chapter 8 ends with a discussion regarding caring for those who self-harm.

In closing I would like to emphasize that this book is not an attempt to answer all the questions there are about suicide-related behaviour. It is, I hope, an attempt to explore some issues that I feel are important in the study of a very human and emotional topic. In raising and discussing these issues I hope to generate debate among students as to how suicide-related behaviour should be addressed in the future.

Columba McLaughlin PhD BSc RNT RN

A personal reflection on suicide-related behaviour

1

The term 'suicide-related behaviour' is a very general term and is used in this book in the belief that it includes all self-inflicted life-threatening behaviours in which a person intended either to harm or kill him or herself and which could, whether intentional or not, result in the person's death. For example, most practitioners will easily place attempted suicide within the concept of suicide-related behaviour. However, there might be differences of opinion as to the inclusion of self-harm within the concept of suicide-related behaviour. In even a brief analysis of the literature, readers will find that while some authors suggest that attempted suicide and self-harm are the same, other authors believe that they are different entities. In this book both self-harm and attempted suicide will be considered as separate entities and differences between both behaviours will be explored and discussed. In addition, having some understanding of the differences between self-harm and attempted suicide will be useful when caring responses and therapeutic approaches to care are considered later on in this book.

This chapter focuses specifically on my own personal reflections on tragic events that on some occasions ended in suicide. The events described are in the form of brief case vignettes, most of which are based on real people and to whom I feel privileged that they allowed me to share their innermost thoughts. Suicide-related behaviour is multi-faceted and the case vignettes outlined here offer only a brief insight into the different ways that the phenomenon of suicide-related behaviour presents itself. For me, each case vignette represents a person's experience of events that have caused distress in them. Each of these people has helped me to focus my professional and academic studies towards people in crisis who have exhibited suicide-related behaviour in one form or another.

Experiencing suicide – a shattered innocence

During adolescence I was involved with two different groups of teenagers. One group was from an urban area and the other was from a rural area. Both groups consisted of teenagers from varying social backgrounds. While both groups mixed well together on many occasions, in general we were most loyal to our primary group. My recollection of that time was that we were a gregarious bunch of young teenagers. Friendships that were formed at that time in our lives have remained since.

However, in our late teens and early twenties on separate occasions three of our friends killed themselves. Each of these suicides shocked us all in both our groups. For all of us these were our first encounters with suicide. Those of us who had heard of the term suicide assumed that it was linked only with mental illness. Others within both groups had never heard of the term until they met it head on. We all knew that each of our friends had no history of mental illness. Each of them had achieved well in college, was in steady employment and each was expected to do well in the future. Then why should they have killed themselves? We came to the conclusion that they had killed themselves as a direct result of ongoing relationship difficulties at the time. We found it hard to believe that they could not find other options to their difficulties other than to take their own lives. The impact of their suicides still remains with me to this day.

Case vignette 1

While I was a newly qualified staff nurse in a busy acute admission ward in a psychiatric hospital, I met and cared for a young person called 'Pat'. On admission to the ward, Pat was detained under the then Mental Health Act for Northern Ireland (1972). Pat was in his late teens and he had a recent history of cutting his wrists. During the handover report on the ward, we were told that Pat was suicidal. As a result of this the joint nursing-medical care plan specified that he be cared for in an open single room and that nursing staff were to observe him every fifteen minutes. Initially, Pat did not communicate nor was he willing to communicate with any of the ward staff. On my turn for observations I found this lack of communication quite difficult to deal with. Nonetheless, I ensured, through a very one-sided form of communication, that he knew that I was there and interested in him.

However, one day another nurse informed me that Pat had somehow managed to obtain a razor blade and had succeeded in cutting his wrists before staff could intervene to stop him. He used half the razor blade, which was removed. Pat's wounds were dressed and efforts were made to find out why he had cut his wrists.

Pat did not offer any explanation. In fact he was very annoyed that he was 'caught in the act'. I recall a member of staff saying that he must have been only 'seeking attention'. Another member of staff commented that the cuts were only scratches, were not life-threatening and if a 'fuss' was made of Pat, it might encourage him to do the same in the future. Regardless of these thoughts, I remember thinking at that time that there were easier and less painful ways of gaining attention from other people.

A search of Pat's room did not reveal where the other half of the razor blade was. Pat was subsequently put on 'Special Observation', which entailed a nurse being with him 24 hours per day. Nurses were instructed to engage Pat in conversation. One aim of this was to find the second half of the razor blade and the second aim was to elicit why Pat cut his wrists. From my own point of view, I found it much easier to communicate with Pat on this occasion as we had the wrist-cutting incident to refer to. This close encounter combined with verbal engagement enabled the nursing staff to break through the communication barrier. On the third day of continuous observation, Pat revealed where the second half of the razor blade was.

Following this incident, Pat and I had a number of discussions and I found that he had quite a few personal difficulties in his life, of which physical abuse, relationship difficulties within his immediate family and alcohol misuse were prominent. However, while he had social and relationship difficulties, he had no history of mental illness and he did not receive a diagnostic label. In our conversations he told me that the first time he had cut himself, his intention had been to die. However, he did not die and he got a feeling of relief after cutting himself. Since then he has never at any time considered suicide as an option. The fact that Pat would willingly cut his wrists but have no wish to die made me curious about the way the human mind thinks and the way we as humans can behave when experiencing psychological pain. It is relevant at this point to mention that Shneidman (1993, p. 51) wrote that 'suicide is caused by psychache' and he also defined psychache as 'psychological pain, in the mind'. However, some 15 years earlier than Shneidman's (1993) book, it had already occurred to me that in some way Pat was using what is now known as self-harm as a method of dealing or coping with his own psychache or emotional despair.

Case vignette 2

Although Marie had several admissions to hospital, I never met her there. She came to my attention through my interactions with professional colleagues working in non-statutory (voluntary) services. Marie had six-year history of self-harm. She had numerous cuts on different parts of her body but her arms bore the bulk of the physical scarring. From the first time that I met her, I found her very pleasant and easy to relate and talk to. At times she was angry at the way some practitioners had treated her in the past but she countered that by saying that on occasion she met well-intentioned practitioners as well. Marie had a horrendous story to tell of sexual, physical and emotional abuse from early childhood until her teenage years. While she was being abused, she believed that the abuse was brought on by herself and that she was responsible for it. Also, she felt that she was alone, trapped and that help was unavailable.

Her initial response to these difficulties in her life was a vague attempt to die. At that time she did not know whether she wanted to live or die. When she was 13 years of age she found the psychological pain of it all too hard to bear. In a frenzy she found a bottle, broke it and used it to cut her arms. At that time she recalled thinking that she did not care whether she lived or died. On this first behavioural response to the abuse, she thought that it was probably a lack of anatomical knowledge that saved her life. However, she did observe that while she felt very tense prior to cutting herself, she felt immense relief once she had done so. In a very similar way this resembled Pat's thinking. Marie began to use self-harm as a way of relieving her psychache.

Marie told me that when her parents realized that she was cutting herself, they took her to her general practitioner (GP) who then had her admitted to hospital. She was the youngest person on the ward and found it difficult to relate to anyone. While in hospital she was diagnosed as having a personality disorder, but did not find this out until later. However, she attributed the way she was treated in hospital to this diagnosis having been attached to her. She did not think that she had a disorder in her personality. She knew that she had difficulties in her life but did not know how to cope with them. She did not know who to trust or who she could talk to. The only effective relief she had until that point was her self-harming behaviour and while in hospital she was deprived of that. She felt that rather than helping her, hospitalization was abusing her all over again. Also, she felt that the establishment of any trusting relationships with those practitioners who seemed helpful was waylaid by the negative attitudes and actions of practitioners who she felt were less than helpful.

On discharge from hospital Marie started to cut her upper body and arms in an effort to hide her self-harming behaviour. Nonetheless, being young she was eventually found out. Over the course of several admissions, Marie's self-harming behaviour did not decrease as she obtained much needed comfort from cutting herself. In her view most practitioners seemed more interested in her self-harming behaviour rather than in her as a person. Also, she felt that no one wanted to address the psychache she was experiencing or the reasons behind it. After several admissions Marie got the impression that most staff did not take her seriously, viewed her as an attention-seeker or as manipulative. At one point she felt that others thought she was a lost cause.

In her teens, the abuse stopped. She felt that this was because she was now older, able to verbalize her complaints and that the perpetrator feared legal action. However, the memories of the abuse remained with her and she still found emotional relief from cutting herself. Thus, her self-harming behaviour continued. In her late teens she met a practitioner who did not diagnose her, was non-judgemental, was interested in her as a person and who helped her unravel and come to terms with the emotions she was experiencing. Currently, Marie lives with a partner; they have two children and she has commenced studies for mature students. In the future she wants to become a counsellor and to help others who have histories of suicide-related behaviour.

Case vignette 3

Sarah was in her late forties when I first met her. She and I met as a direct result of research that I was involved with. Sarah was married and had several teenage children. She had a history of suicide-related behaviour, which resulted in over ten admissions to hospital. Her case notes revealed that she had a diagnosis of borderline personality disorder, a long history of alcohol abuse and – as mentioned in her case notes – deliberate self-harm by overdosing on prescribed medication. On this occasion, Sarah had been admitted to a casualty department following another overdose of prescribed medication. Subsequently, she was transferred to the local psychiatric hospital. The medical opinion was that Sarah had low self-esteem as a result of alcohol abuse and that she was in danger of harming or killing herself.

The medical opinion did not tell the whole of Sarah's story. In general, Sarah, although impulsive in her behaviour at times, was really quite shy. I mentioned this to other staff but they were of the view that Sarah used this shyness to manipulate other people and that that would include me. Nonetheless, I found her open about her past history and I took an empathic non-judgemental approach when communicating with her. Sarah told me about her relationship with her husband. From what she told me it was a brutal and violent marriage in which she was much abused over many years. She was quite graphic in her details of the abuse. She felt trapped in that she felt that she could not leave home as the children were too young and she did not know where to go. In addition, Sarah feared that her husband would have followed her and that this could have disastrous consequences for her and the children. I asked her about her harming herself through overdosing. She told me that initially and on some occasions she had thought of killing herself but most times her intention was to get some sleep, obtain rest and to get away from the abuse. I also asked her about her alcohol abuse. She admitted to having a problem with alcohol but she felt that alcohol was a coping measure and a great release to her. It numbed the psychological pain of the distress she was experiencing. In addition, she felt that if the abuse was resolved, then she would be able to deal with the alcohol problem. Sarah made one statement that has always remained with me and that was 'My doctor doesn't understand why I drink.'

Although I was not directly involved in Sarah's care programme, I did ask her permission to share what she told me with practitioners who had responsibility for her care. This she agreed to on condition that I passed the information on to specific practitioners who she thought were helpful and could be trusted. This I was very happy to do. These practitioners, in agreement with Sarah, adjusted her care programme to involve specific therapy that would address negative aspects in her life such as the physical and sexual abuse she had experienced in the past.

Case vignette 4

Stephen was admitted to a casualty department after being found unconscious at his home. He smelt of alcohol and the person who found him felt that he may also have taken an overdose as an empty bottle of paracetamol was found beside him. Whilst in casualty he was given an emetic to induce vomiting and the remains of the paracetamol tablets were found in the regurgitated gastric contents. In our opinion he was very lucky to be alive.

Stephen and his partner Joan had been living together for three years. Both had decided to settle in Joan's home town. This resulted in Stephen having to move several hundred miles from his home town. They had invested in a new home, which took all of Stephen's monthly income and almost half of Joan's monthly income to meet the mortgage repayments. Such a financial burden led to both partners working as much overtime as possible. Unfortunately, this arrangement played havoc on the amount of time they spent in each other's company. Over several months, both Stephen and Joan had a number of disagreements, all of which seem to revolve around financial matters and how much time they spent together. Stephen still loved Joan but did not know how to resolve the financial and other pressures that they were facing.

One evening Stephen came home early from work and he found Joan in a compromising position with another man. An argument ensued, during which she said that she wanted to end the relationship and that he could keep both the house and the mortgage. She then moved out to live with this man. In Stephen's evaluation he had been deserted by the person he loved, was left with a substantial financial burden and he felt isolated as his family lived 200 miles away. He did not know what to do. On opening a cupboard in the kitchen he found a bottle of whisky and beside it a bottle containing paracetamol tablets. He took both bottles and sat down on the settee in the living room. His thinking at that moment was to die and he felt that if he drank enough whisky it would dull the pain of swallowing the tablets. In effect, Stephen's suicidal thinking was a direct result of a breakdown in the relationship with his girlfriend.

Fortunately for Stephen a neighbour had seen his partner leave in a hurry and with a stranger and assumed that there had been an argument. This neighbour noticed no movement about the house and decided to call over just to see how Stephen was. When he received no answer after ringing the doorbell, he began looking in the windows. On seeing Stephen in a collapsed state he tried to waken Stephen by knocking on the window. On being unable to waken Stephen, the neighbour called the police and an ambulance.

In casualty the next morning, we met Stephen and we found that he felt embarrassed about the whole incident. Initially he was very reluctant to talk, but he eventually began to describe the events that lead up to his taking an overdose. At the time he took the tablets, his intention was to die. In fact he scored very high on the items in the Suicide Intent Scale as described by Beck, Schuyler and Herman (1974). However, at this moment he no longer felt that way and was glad to be alive. Stephen was offered crisis counselling rather than admission to hospital. After several sessions he felt well enough to deal with the aftermath of the break up of the relationship and to get on with his life. Following the sale of his house, Stephen moved back to his home town, his family, old friends and a new job.

Case vignette 5

Elizabeth was a married lady in her early seventies. During their lives together, she and her husband had got on very well. They had two daughters and several grandchildren. While in her sixties, Elizabeth had been treated by her GP for depression and had made a good recovery. Recently, she had been suffering from tiredness and she also had an arthritic pain in her left hip. One Saturday afternoon she was feeling poorly and she took some of her prescribed analgesia and went to bed. She suggested to her husband that he should go and visit the family of Jean, their oldest daughter. However, when the husband arrived at Jean's house, Jean suggested that they all go to visit their mother and grandmother. On arrival at her mother's house Jean found her mother in a collapsed state in the bath with a serious laceration to her left wrist. Elizabeth had used a bread knife to inflict the wound, which was so severe that it necessitated her being rushed to theatre for surgery to repair the Ulnar Artery and to have tendon and nerves repaired.

Early the next morning, my mentor telephoned me and asked me to meet her in the casualty department to assess Elizabeth. When we met Elizabeth she was not pleased to see us and she made this very clear when she said that she wanted to meet St Peter rather than us. She wanted to be dead and had no wish to meet her husband, daughter or any other member of her family. She blamed the knife and said that it must have been blunt. We allowed Elizabeth to express her emotions and eventually she reluctantly began to tell what happened. In our assessment we found that although she was treated for depression by her GP eight years earlier, she had had no contact with the mental health services since. She had a very successful life, had a loving family and was very secure in her elderly years. Why did Elizabeth want to die? She did not relish the thought of getting old and wanted to die at a time that suited her. She did not want to become a burden on her family nor on anyone else. She had made her peace with God and believed that St Peter would understand her motives. It took most of the day for us to convince Elizabeth to talk to her immediate family. They, while being shocked at her attempted suicide, encouraged her to seek voluntary admission to hospital. Elizabeth agreed to this. During her time in hospital, Elizabeth took part in Cognitive Behavioural Therapy. Meanwhile, her husband and daughters sought advice on aftercare following discharge. After several weeks of in-hospital care, Elizabeth was discharged home with follow-up support from a Cognitive Behavioural Psychotherapist.

Case vignette 6

When I first met John he was withdrawn, spoke very little, looked very sad and very lethargic. John had been admitted to hospital on several previous occasions. John was in his late forties and was a successful businessman. Also, he had a loving wife and several grown-up children who were now adults. His family were very concerned about him and they visited him regularly. John had been diagnosed as suffering from clinical depression. On this occasion he was very depressed and had expressed suicide-related ideation. His GP and his immediate family were concerned that John might have killed himself. For these reasons, John was admitted to the ward.

Communicating or connecting with John was very difficult. However, we had no choice but to ensure that John knew that we were available and willing to listen to him. We did this because we were concerned about the possibility of his killing himself. Even though John had no previous history of suicide-related behaviour, the fact that he had previously expressed it to his GP meant that it must be explored. However, he denied any such thoughts about harming or killing himself. In addition, the nursing interactions with John and the observations made on his behaviour and his interactions with others did not suggest any suicidal thoughts. In fact, during his time in hospital, at no time did John ever express any intention of suicide and subsequently he was considered at low risk of suicide.

During the course of his in-hospital treatment, John's medication was reviewed and the consultant ordered a course of Electro Convulsive Therapy. In time John became more active, took more interest in his surroundings and in himself and he began to communicate more with staff. On one occasion when his mood was showing improvement he was asked about his depression. However, he was unable to give an explanation as to why he felt the way he did. He knew all about the good and positive things in his life but these did not connect with him nor did they ease his depressive feelings. For some reason unknown to himself and indeed to others, he just could not be bothered about anything during the time he felt so depressed. However, John made steady progress, his mood improved and his interactions and relationships with his family also improved. Weekend leave was encouraged and John also began to take an interest in his business again. Eventually, John was discharged into the care of his GP and the Community Psychiatric Team. Approximately four months later, we heard that John had killed himself. All of the staff on the ward were shocked and we never found out why he had done so.

Summary

I have deliberately begun this book with a personal reflection of these case vignettes because each of them has created in me powerful emotions that made me aware of myself first as a human being and secondly as a professional. Each of the suicides created an apprehension in me at the time and they still do today as I reflect on these past events. Similarly, a curiosity was created in me regarding the care required by people in psychological crisis. In addition, I became very curious about trying to understand the relationship between self-harm and suicide. No matter which way one views each case vignette, in each there is the potential, whether intentional or not, for death by one's own hand. In addition, in my professional journey to date I have met numerous people who have been bereaved by suicide. To this day, while many have managed to come to terms and accept what has happened, none has recovered fully from the loss. It remains my belief that suicide provokes powerful emotions in all those who have come to experience it through the loss of family or friends and that these emotions are long-lasting.

As a direct result of my experiences and in trying to understand the human mind and why humans behave the way they do when under duress, I began to study psychology. The combination of mental health nursing and psychology created in me a lifelong interest in trying to understand and care for people in psychological crisis who harm or try to kill themselves.

Contemporary issues in suicide-related behaviour

2

In Chapter 2 a number of contemporary issues are explored. These are:

1. Suicide-related behaviour – the ultimate contradiction
2. Ethical issues in suicide-related behaviour
3. Rational suicide
4. Euthanasia
5. Legal and religious issues
6. Attitudes to suicide-related behaviour
7. Attitudes of 'others' to suicidal behaviour
8. Competency in interpersonal skills

Suicide-related behaviour – the ultimate contradiction

Asking practitioners to accept that suicide or any suicide-related behaviour is an optional behaviour for some people and in some cases there is a possibility that suicide may be the right decision and then asking practitioners to prevent future suicide is asking a lot. Both requests are contradictory to each other and also poles apart. In fact suicide is a contradiction in terms. For example, Nietzsche once said that 'It is always consoling to think of suicide; in that way one gets through many a bad night.' This is a very contradictory statement and suggests that thinking about suicide is one way of helping a person to cope with some stressor that is causing them mental angst. In addition, Nietzsche also commented that 'when one does away with oneself one does the most estimable thing possible: one thereby almost deserves to live'. In a way, Nietzsche is saying that suicide is an admirable act, yet it causes so much suffering to those who are left behind! In reality, whether practitioners agree or not, suicide does offer the person a permanent and final release from their deep psychological pain. Yet in achieving that permanent release, the person is not alive to appreciate the newfound peace of mind. In suicide, the very mind that sought peace has been destroyed by the means it used to obtain the peace. Because of this, a number of authors and philosophers have called suicide the ultimate contradiction.

The thought of suicide has crossed the minds of many people. For example, during 2005 in the United Kingdom and the Republic of Ireland the Samaritans recorded approximately 474 000 calls where people stated that they were feeling suicidal at that particular moment (Samaritans, 2006). In the islands of Ireland and Great Britain that number is equivalent to one person contemplating suicide every minute of every day during 2005. In addition, I can recall a conference in the North of England (UK) in late 2003 in which Professor Philip Barker, the keynote speaker, asked some 200 delegates, 'Hands up how many of you have ever considered killing yourselves?' For some reason I was not surprised when most of the delegates put their hands up. To the minority who did not put their hands up he asked, 'Why not? Have you no imagination?' It is important that mental health practitioners realize that many people in crisis do think of suicide as an option and in many cases people believe that suicide works. Whether we as practitioners agree or not, suicide is popular as an effective and very permanent end to psychache. For example, during 2002 in the United Kingdom of Great Britain and Northern Ireland, according to the Office of National Statistics, the General Register Office (Scotland) and the Northern Ireland Statistics and Research Agency, there were a total of 5857 deaths recorded as suicides and undetermined deaths. That is equivalent to a rate of 12.14 per 100 000 in those aged 15 years and over. Put another way that is one suicide almost every two hours, or almost 113 suicides per week in the United Kingdom. Also, according to the Central Statistics Office (Republic of Ireland) and the Northern Ireland Statistics and Research Agency, during 2002 on the island of Ireland there were a total of 638 recorded suicides, which is equivalent to 14.48 per 100 000 population in those aged 15 years and older. Put another way, approximately 12 people will kill themselves each week on the island of Ireland.

The perceived reason why a person would consider killing himself and the reaction of family and friends add to the contradiction. For example, during wartime if a soldier sacrifices his own life to save colleagues or for the greater good of their community, they are frequently deemed a hero. Such suicides are examples of Durkheim's (1897/1951) 'altruistic suicide'. For instance, during the Second World War, many young Japanese pilots placed their sense of duty to their emperor and to their country higher than their own personal welfare. In doing so they welded themselves into their explosive-filled aircraft and then killed themselves by dive-bombing and crashing their planes into the allied warships. The term used for this act was 'Kamikaze'. Literally, this term means 'Divine Wind'. In more recent times there have been similar acts in the Middle East conflict. For instance the 'suicide-bomber' is seen as a terrorist by one set of combatants; however, they are seen as heroes or heroines by their own side. Whether or not we agree about the legitimacy of these (suicide) acts, it appears from pre-recorded video tapes of the person that they were committed to their ideals and what they were about to do. Also, the acts of 11 September 2001, when hijacked airplanes were deliberately crashed into New York's Twin Towers, resulting in the deaths of almost 3000 innocent lives, fall into this category. There is a possibility that some of these persons may have been coerced; however, many will have set out knowing that they were not going to survive and for a cause which they believed in. These acts of suicide are frequently seen, by groups of people within a culture, as being acceptable and appropriate while people from another culture may strongly disagree and see them as terrorist acts. The main controversy that arises here is that other people, who are innocent victims, are killed alongside the suicide-bomber. Nonetheless, all of the above examples of suicide have 'duty' to a greater cause as an underlying belief. However, one type of wartime suicide that conforms to Durkheim's altruistic suicide is that of the soldier who sacrifices his own life in order that his comrades will live. This type of act is deemed as a mark of heroism with the ultimate sacrifice for the greater good.

In what seems like a total contradiction to this latter reason, the Japanese act of *hara-kiri* is a culturally accepted form of ritualistic suicide that is performed to save face, atone for bringing shame to the family or group, or to protect the honour of the person, family or group. For example, *hara-kiri* was one way in which a defeated or captured Japanese Samurai could redeem his honour. Frequently, the act of *hara-kiri* would involve disembowelment by one's own sword. This act was drawn out over a lengthy period of time and more often than not the person had a friend stand by who would decapitate them and end their suffering. Another culturally acceptable form of suicide in Japanese culture was that of *seppuku*. This is a form of *hara-kiri* in which the act of suicide was the same but the term was reserved for nobility who were condemned to death. In effect, the act of *seppuku* saved the noble person the spectacle of a public death as a common criminal. Thus, the broad reasons why people would kill themselves can vary from being altruistic and for the common good or to save face or public humiliation. However, in contrast, in the Western hemisphere a person who kills himself to avoid a conviction for a criminal offence or family scandal is sometimes seen as being cowardly. Thus, it seems that suicide is more acceptable by one group of people and for some specific reasons and yet is not acceptable by other groups.

Also, the way in which a person carries out the suicide is frequently controversial. For example, rarely is suicide or any related behaviour carried out in the public view. One could argue that jumping off a high building would be in the public view. This is true but the numbers of people who kill themselves by jumping off high buildings is much lower than the number of people who kill themselves by hanging or by poisoning. More often than not the act of suicide is usually a very private action for the person. Frequently, the person is alone when they harm or kill themselves and usually it may be some time before their body is found. However, in total contradiction to the loneliness of the person at the time of the suicide, the impact of the suicide on practitioners and other people, especially family and friends, is very public and intense. Frequently, the person may have left a note that says that they do not want to hurt a particular family member or close friend. However, their suicide can frequently have the opposite effect, as the family member may feel responsible for the person's death.

During crisis the person may have difficulty in finding a solution. At this point he (she) may consider suicide-related behaviour where the intention is either to harm him (her) self or to end his (her) life. This is another contradiction and is in direct contrast to the aims of health professionals whose job it is to repair physical harm and to maintain life. With these contrasting aims how can a practitioner help someone who is trying to harm him (her) self or trying to end their life? While in the caring environment we often assume that the person is a willing partner in their own care and that they are willing to negotiate the care necessary to help them return to normality. This type of contradiction can place the practitioner at odds with the person who is in despair and vice versa. Emotions can become intense as each does battle to meet their own aim. This type of contradiction is very similar to that I felt when I first met Pat in the acute admission ward (see Chapter 1). He had been admitted to hospital after his family had found out that he was cutting his wrists. Senior staff told me that Pat was suicidal. However, in discussion with him I found out that his aim was not to die by suicide but to ease his psychache by harming himself. In the initial stages, the health care team's aim was to prevent Pat from doing further harm to himself and to prevent him from killing himself. Thus, in the early stages of Pat's care the qualified staff in the ward were on a collision course with Pat as their aims for his care were contradictory to Pat's aims.

Suicide and its related behaviour are contradictory and contentious in their nature and it is this that gives rise to intense emotions in practitioners and in the people who need relief from their psychache. Some people are so focused on their self-harming behaviour or planning their actual suicide that they have difficulty in contemplating any other behavioural option. In contrast, practitioners in their quest to help people recover and rebuild or repair their lives are frequently in a position to identify a number of feasible options. At such times, practitioners may find themselves in a dilemma as to whether or not to reveal these options. To impose these options without the person's agreement could very likely defeat the purpose of therapy. Certainly, not only is there a contradiction here but there is also potential conflict between the person and practitioners. When it comes to suicide-related behaviour, practitioners would be well advised to consider some of these contradictory areas in relation to their own beliefs. In doing so they may open previously closed doors between themselves and the person who is experiencing psychache.

Ethical issues in suicide-related behaviour

All of us will agree that every person who is living on this planet has at least one lifetime event in common with everyone else. This event is that we will all die at some time. The main difference between people is how each of us will die. However, most practitioners will agree that we should never have to commit suicide. Also, I am sure that most practitioners have at some stage asked themselves one or both of the following questions: (1) Is there ever a reason for suicide-related behaviour? (2) Is any form of suicide-related behaviour ever the right thing to do? It would be quite right to assume that for some people there are reasons and there are times when suicide-related behaviour is the right thing to do. However, for other people, there is never a time when suicide-related behaviour is the right thing to do. Thus, there are two opposing viewpoints.

Discussion points: In a small group (no more than six students), spend 10–15 minutes discussing whether or not any form of suicide-related behaviour is ever or never the right thing to do. Make sure that you include rationale for your decisions. Write down some notes on your decisions and compare these notes with other groups.

Case vignette 7

Consider Bridget's brief case history. From about the age of 6 years a male family member sexually abused Bridget. Over the years this caused her great distress. She found that she could not escape from it. She had no one to go to or to talk to. She felt she could not trust her teachers at school. In reality she felt alone. Eventually she developed feelings of despair and one evening, when she was 13 years of age, she felt that she could take no more and decided to kill herself. She used a broken piece of glass to cut one of her wrists. The pain of cutting was severe but fortunately for her, the wounds were superficial. However, she felt emotionally relieved by the act. To hide her scars from her parents she wore long sleeves. However, because of the emotional relief she experienced she carried on cutting, a less obvious part of her body, until she was 19 years old.

Discussion points: In a small group of fellow students, spend 10–15 minutes discussing your thoughts about Bridget's suicide-related behaviour. If you were aged 13 and in her position, what would you have done? What (realistic) alternatives did she have? Why do you think that these alternatives might succeed?

Case vignette 8

Consider the case of Mike. This case has been reported in a national daily paper in Great Britain (Mackinnon, 2005). Even so a pseudonym is still used here to offer Mike some form of protection. Mike was a 14-year-old schoolboy who was being bullied at school. Other pupils attacked him on his way to and from school. Bullies damaged his books and even his bicycle. At mealtimes the bullies threw food at him. When he took the bus to and from school he was attacked at the bus stop and even on the bus. On one occasion his tormentors used a mobile telephone to film him being bullied. This was then sent to other pupils. Eventually his parents took the matter up with the school authorities who arranged a meeting between staff, Mike and the bully. However, during the meeting Mike was verbally abused by the bully again. His parents moved him from the school but the bullying recommenced at the new school. Although Mike was tall for his age and bigger than those who were bullying him, he refused to strike back at any of them. The bullying drove Mike to cut his wrists and to think very seriously about suicide. On one occasion his parents caught Mike looking at Internet sites showing people how to hang themselves.

Discussion points: In a small group of fellow students spend 10–15 minutes discussing your thoughts about Mike's suicide-related behaviour. If you were in his position, what would you have done? What (realistic) alternatives did he have? Why do you think that these alternatives might succeed?

In all of the behaviours associated with suicide, the most controversial is suicide itself. Why is this? Well, it is possible to offer some form of rationale that explains why a person may want to harm rather than kill themselves or have any thoughts about suicide. Such explanations can range from self-inflicted punishment, emotional relief or the intention of inducing high sexual arousal in the person. However, controversy can and does arise when it is known that a person died as a direct result of his or her own behaviour. Key ethical issues here still revolve around the two same issues: (1) having a reason to die by one's own hand and (2) having a right to die by one's own hand.

In most religious belief systems killing another person is deemed as wrong and the term murder is used to describe it. Some professionals would equate suicide with the term self-murder and therefore it could be argued that suicide is wrong both morally and legally. For example, for many years attempted suicide was classified as a misdemeanour and punishable by law in both Great Britain and in Northern Ireland. In Britain there were a number of successful prosecutions (Keir, 1986). However, the Suicide Act (1961) in Great Britain and the Criminal Justice Act (1966) in Northern Ireland established that it was no longer a misdemeanour. But, is suicide wrong in all cases? Let us look at a few prominent examples.

Case vignette 9

The acts of *Hara-kiri* and *Seppuku* have been mentioned earlier. One could argue that these acts are remnants of Japan's militaristic past. However, in November 1970, Yukio Mishima, one of Japan's most famous postwar writers killed himself with an act of *hara-kiri*. In that year, in an attempt to get Japan to return to its militaristic past, Mishima and other colleagues kidnapped a Japanese army general. They then demanded that the soldiers in his command hear a speech by Mishima that was designed to get them to revolt against the government and to defend and restore the power of the Emperor. Unfortunately, the soldiers jeered and laughed at him. Immediately, Mishima stepped into the building and proceeded with the ritualistic act of *hara-kiri*. One of his assistants (eventually) ended his suffering by decapitating him. While there is evidence that Mishima had prepared for the act of *hara-kiri*, his reasons why he did so may not be so clear. For example, his death could have been interpreted as a demonstration of his loyalty towards his ideals and his Emperor. Alternatively, it may be that for Mishima not to have killed himself would have been an act of shame or humiliation.

Discussion points: In a small group of fellow students spend 10–15 minutes discussing your thoughts about Mishima's suicide. Should he have killed himself? What (realistic) alternatives did he have? What rationale do you have for your conclusion?

Case vignette 10

In April 1994, Kurt Cobain, lead singer in the rock band Nirvana, was found dead in his home. He had a single gunshot to the head and there was a gun and a suicide note nearby. The content of the note suggests that Kurt had not been experiencing the excitement of performing or of creating music for a number of years and that the worst crime he could think of would be to 'rip people off by faking it and pretending as if I'm having 100% fun'. At one point in the note Kurt writes, 'the sad little sensitive, unappreciative Pisces, Jesus man. Why don't you just enjoy it? I don't know!' In his suicide note he also wrote, 'it's better to burn out than to fade away'. Moreover, in his final sentence he asked his wife (Courtney Love) to keep going for their daughter Frances for her life would be better without him. His final written words were in large capital letters – I LOVE YOU, I LOVE YOU. This note is in the public domain and was available to view when I checked it on 16 November 2006 on the World Wide Web: http://www.justiceforkurt. com/investigation/documents/note_scan.shtml. However, web site addresses do change or close down and should this happen to the above web site address, you can access it by following links to Kurt Cobain's death.

The suicide note provides a deep insight into the inner conflict that Kurt Cobain had been experiencing. There is a difference between Kurt's suicide and Mishima's *hara-kiri*. The suicide of Mishima seems to have been affected by external events. However, in Kurt Cobain's case it seems that he was wrestling with his own inner conflicts. In addition, Kurt apparently had had enough of psych-ache and emotional despair. Some might say: why didn't he just get on and enjoy his fame? However, Kurt had already asked that question in his note. Unfortunately, he did not have an answer.

Discussion points: In a small group of fellow students, spend 10–15 minutes discussing your thoughts about Kurt Cobain's suicide. Should he have killed himself? What (realistic) alternatives did he have? What rationale do you have for your conclusion?

Case vignette 11

In addition, in February 2006 it was reported in a number of papers and on the World Wide Web that a Gerald ('Gerry') Georgettis was found hanged in the toilet of an airplane. It seems that he hanged himself in mid-flight after he was accused of arson. Gerry Georgettis was famous in that he worked as a sound engineer with a number of famous bands such as Pink Floyd, Red Hot Chilli Peppers and Cold Chisel. He had an international reputation stretching from Australia, to USA and Great Britain. While working as a theatre manager in Miami (USA) he bought a new car from a dealer. However, when he got home he felt that he had been scammed (cheated) in the price he had to pay for the car. He returned to the dealership, drove his new car through the window of the building, poured fuel over it and other cars and set fire to it. There was an estimated $1 million damage done including damage to the building, and 11 cars including his own were destroyed. Also, a limited edition of a Ford GT, one of 250 specially made and a collector's item worth $150 000, was damaged. As there were people in the building Gerry was charged with first degree arson which carried a penalty of up to

30 years in prison. Three days later on a flight from Washington to Los Angeles, Gerry's body was found in the toilet of a plane.

Discussion points: In a small group of fellow students spend 10–15 minutes discussing your thoughts about Gerry's suicide. Should he have killed himself? What (realistic) alternatives did he have? What rationale do you have for your conclusion?

An argument that exists within the realms of reasons for suicide is that of 'what are the alternatives to suicide?' In each of the examples above you were asked for realistic alternative behaviours that could replace the suicide-related behaviour. Now would be a good time for you to list the alternatives that your group came up with. A conclusion that you may have drawn is that suicide would be inappropriate when other behaviours were available that could have resolved the person's life difficulties and reduced the person's feelings of despair.

In discussing the above examples you will now have some thoughts about whether there are ever sufficient reasons for suicide. However, at this point it would be useful to consider whether or not suicide is ever the right thing to do. For instance, it is important to realize that when people harm themselves and the family finds out about this behaviour, concerns and anxieties may increase within the family. Sometimes parents and other family members may be adversely affected by the behaviour of their retative. Thus, suicide-related behaviour can have an effect not just on the suicidal person but on those around them as well. Similarly, the person who is contemplating suicide will think of his or her own reasons for suicide. They may have some degree of rationale but do they have the right to go ahead with it? As mentioned earlier, suicide does provide a permanent solution to any problem that a person is concerned with. However, the suicide of a person also creates long-lasting emotional difficulties for those family, friends and colleagues left behind. Consider the case of Ray Gomersal who killed himself after his son and daughter both killed themselves (Bone, 2005). He found it difficult coping with the death of his son, but after his daughter's suicide in July, he said that although he would cope, he had nothing to live for. In November 2005 he was found hanged at home (Bone, 2005). Putting it very bluntly, other people within the person's circle of family, friends and colleagues have rights as well. Certainly, any person contemplating suicide and their right to suicide should also consider the feelings and rights of others who are close to them.

Rational suicide

Is there ever such a thing as a rational suicide? Most, if not all, dictionaries and Thesauruses will associate the word rational with other words such as: (1) logical, (2) realistic and (3) based on reason. More often than not, people and in some cases the media, associate suicide with people who are depressed, are not thinking clearly, or are suffering from temporary insanity. The list of such associations goes on but one has to ask, can a person be suicidal, be of sound mind and be rational at the same time? Looking back at the previous examples and discussions, what do think?

Case vignette 12

In exploring the case for a rational suicide, it would be useful at this point to consider the case of Nico Speijer who killed himself in September 1981. What was special about Speijer was that he was a renowned Dutch suicidologist and for most of his professional life he was a major proponent of suicide prevention. However, for a long time he had been suffering from intestinal carcinoma, and metastases had spread throughout his body. He had, on a number of occasions, talked to his wife and his colleagues about his condition. Up until the time of his death he was able to control the pain but then found that he could no longer cope with it. Shortly before his death he wrote a note to Professor Diekstra, his long-time friend and colleague, explaining his reasons for killing himself.

Discussion points: In a small group of fellow students spend 10–15 minutes discussing your thoughts about Speijer's suicide. Was his suicide rational? What is your rationale for your answer? The significance of Speijer's suicide is explored in an article by Diekstra (1986) and may be helpful in your discussions.

Whether or not suicide is ever a rational act is very debatable. Certainly, those persons who are totally opposed to suicide will always argue that suicide is an irrational act. With the exception of some people who are mentally disordered, most people can take responsibility for the way in which they run and live their own lives. Unfortunately, some people in acute mental crisis and those who act impulsively are frequently not in a position to consider alternatives to suicide. In such cases, people can and frequently do produce a rationale for their suicide. However, even when there is a rationale for a suicide, not everyone can argue that their particular suicide is the right thing to do. In conclusion, and to address the two questions that were asked earlier in this chapter, it can be argued that there is a rationale in some suicides but not in all cases. However, when examining whether suicide is ever the right thing to do at any time, it is worth remembering that the rights of others such as family, friends and colleagues are important as well. For instance, the person may permanently resolve their difficulties through suicide, but the suicide may create other difficulties for those left behind. In addition, it is worth considering that the suicide of a person can be a very high price to pay for resolving one of life's difficulties. This is particularly true when there were untried alternatives to suicide available and the person either did not or was not able to access them.

Euthanasia

To die by suicide is not always a nice, clean, happy death. The gunshot wound to the head does not leave a pretty sight. In hanging, the person will frequently defecate and may also urinate either prior to death or at the moment of death. Also, harrowing stories about the act can be heard from those who survive. For budding students it might be very informative for them to get some experience, particularly at the weekend, in the accident and emergency wards of a large inner-city general hospital. However, there are other issues with suicide-related behaviour that make it seem like an unpleasant end to life. For example, the loneliness a person feels when they are in a car in the middle of nowhere and they are trying to poison themselves with carbon monoxide. Or visualize the lonely scene of a person in a bedsit swallowing a cocktail of tablets, cutting their wrists, or setting up the gear necessary to hang themselves. Sometimes it seems that suicide is not a good death. However, in contrast, euthanasia is a term that literally means 'good death'. When a person who is considering suicide thinks through their rationale for their suicide, it may seem much better to have previously sorted out all their earthly issues and then to have someone there with them to provide some form of comfort in their dying moments. Frequently, euthanasia is known as assisted-suicide.

Case vignette 13

The following case is fictionally based and does not refer to any person living or dead. Joseph is a 67-year-old man who has a long history of rheumatoid arthritis. He lives with his wife and they have two sons who are married. Joseph has been confined to a wheelchair for a number of years. However, in recent years he has been diagnosed with bone cancer in his right leg. Metastases have now spread to other parts of his body and he is finding the pain of it intolerable. Recently he has spoken to his wife and family about the possibility of euthanasia. They have decided to ask your opinion.

Discussion point: In a small group of fellow students spend 10–15 minutes discussing how you would respond to the family's request. Write down your rationale for your response.

Euthanasia has been known about for some time. For example, and in my opinion, it was introduced gently to the public in the 1970s film *Logan's Run*. In this film people on reaching the 'ripe old age of 30' are required to present themselves to the authorities so that they can be renewed through a process of death. In addition, in Case vignette 12 above you were asked to discuss the case of Nico Speijer. At this point it is worthwhile noting that while he was an advocate for suicide prevention he, along with his colleague Professor Diekstra, published the first text on assisted-suicide in 1980 (Speijer and Diekstra, 1980). Since then euthanasia has been brought to the attention of the public through the activities of Dr Jack Kevorkian. He was also known as the 'Suicide Doctor' (Kevorkian, 1991). It is well known that Dr Kevorkian had been helping people to die before there were any laws passed making assisted suicide legal. He was convicted in April 1999, at the age of 71, of killing Thomas Youk and was sentenced to 10–25 years in prison. From 1 June 2007 Dr Jack Kevorkian was released from prison.

There are a number of different types of euthanasia. However, there are problems with all forms of it. For example, passive euthanasia is frequently a slow, lengthy process. In general, passive euthanasia involves omitting an act that could save the person's life. For example, in the case of a terminally ill person there might be a medical order not to resuscitate the person if they have a respiratory or cardiac crisis. On the other hand, active euthanasia is an act by a fellow human being that kills a person. Obviously this type of euthanasia could be interpreted as murder. In addition, if a medical doctor performs active euthanasia it would violate their Hippocratic Oath. However, another person does not perform assisted-suicide. In assisted suicide the equipment is made available by which the person can then end their own life. It is not the doctor or other practitioner who will perform the deed, it is the person themselves who will press the button or who will put the mask over their face. Nonetheless, whichever way you look at euthanasia, there are ethical and moral issues that need to be addressed.

Case vignette 14

The following case is fictionally based and does not refer to any person alive or dead. Joan is a 72-year-old female who has been widowed for six years. She has five children who are all in relationships and who have produced 18 grandchildren. Joan has had a history of congestive heart failure and respiratory distress in the last ten years. Also, she has survived a total of eight cardiac arrests. In recent times she has become more breathless and most times she requires the use of a wheelchair to get around. Recently she was admitted to the cardiology unit and then transferred to the medical ward. The medical team have agreed that in the event of another cardiac arrest she is not to be resuscitated and have written DNR (Do Not Resuscitate) in bold letters on the front cover of her case notes. At 3.15 a.m. and while you are in charge on night duty in the medical ward, Joan has a cardiac arrest. What do you do?

Discussion point: In a small group of fellow students spend 10–15 minutes discussing how you would respond to Joan's cardiac arrest. Should you obey the 'do not resuscitate' request or should you ignore it? Write down your rationale for your action.

The legalities of euthanasia have certainly been considered by some USA states. For example, Washington and California have both considered it but these failed when referenda were held. However, in 1994 the state of Oregon became the first American state to allow a doctor to prescribe drugs that would be explicitly used for the suicide of a person. This law was first legally enacted in Oregon in 1998 when an elderly lady with cancer became the first person to legally die with the assistance of a doctor. In effect, Oregon had passed a law that allows doctors to assist in suicide. Elsewhere, such a law had been operating in Holland since 1993. In this law there are safeguards but Maris, Berman and Silverman (2000) highlight potential abuses of the law. One of the most important potential abuses was that it seemed that the doctors had too much power regarding the final decision. Decisions that are solely based on a medical perspective may be flawed. For example, a study reported by Suarez-Almazor *et al.* (2002) suggests that while 69% (n = 100) of people with terminal cancer supported euthanasia in some particular cases, the views expressed were primarily based on psychosocial traits and beliefs rather than on the person's medical symptoms. Thus, it seems that medical personnel should not make decisions about euthanasia without considering the person's feelings as well. In addition, in the United Kingdom (UK) a study carried out by Dickinson *et al.* (2002) found that 80% of geriatricians and 52% of intensive care doctors thought that euthanasia was never justified. They concluded that it would be difficult to legalize euthanasia in the UK unless doctors were certain that appropriate safeguards were in place. Similarly, Essinger (2003) reported that 47% of physicians would oppose the legalization of euthanasia or physician assisted suicide. In addition, the majority of physicians agreed on safeguards and restrictions to protect vulnerable people and to prevent any abuse. Nonetheless, the genie is well and truly out of the bottle and a time could come when euthanasia may be considered as an option in the future.

For practitioners the main issues in euthanasia are very similar to those in suicide. Both actions bring about the premature death of the person. In both cases the questions revolve around (1) the rationality of the suicide or the euthanasia and (2) whether the suicide or euthanasia is the right thing to do. The main difference between the two is that in suicide, the act is usually a lonely one. However, in euthanasia another person would be involved and therefore could provide some form of comfort in the dying moments. With people suffering unrelenting and terminal pain, should we as professionals not help them to die in peace and with dignity? Certainly Maris, Berman and Silverman (2000, p. 469) state their case very clearly when they write, 'Sometimes we need to die, not be kept alive pointlessly – and we deserve to be helped to die in such circumstances.' This statement is very poignant and coming from such eminent authors the subject of euthanasia is worthy of further consideration by practitioners.

Legal and religious issues

For many years negative attitudes to suicide and its related behaviour were upheld by legislation and by religious doctrines. In Great Britain, attempted suicide was a misdemeanour and punishable by law until 1961. Also in Great Britain, during and at the end of the nineteenth century attempted suicide was seen as attempted murder and on occasion was punished by hanging. Also, there were a number of successful prosecutions in the early part of the twentieth century (Keir, 1986). However, the Suicide Act (1961) in Great Britain and the Criminal Justice Act (1966) in Northern Ireland established that it was no longer a misdemeanour. Suicide and attempted suicide are no longer offences. In 1993, the Republic of Ireland was the last European country to decriminalize suicide by the Criminal Law (Suicide) Act. While suicide is not illegal in any state within the United States of America, according to Leenaars and Connolly (2001) there are some variations and some states currently have penalties for those that attempt suicide.

Also, while the Old Testament did not prohibit suicide, both the Christian and Jewish faiths have since considered suicide as being wrong. The Christian faith holds that suicide is a sin and breaks the sixth commandment. In addition, individuals who attempted suicide were also classified as sinners with the possibility of excommunication from the Church. With such strict laws in the Church and the general thought among the public that suicide was a sin, it is no wonder that many of those who died by suicide were buried outside of consecrated ground. Frequently these graves were at crossroads so that every beggar's foot might tramp upon them (Keir, 1986). However some changes came about as different views emerged during and after the religious Reformation. Currently, churches seem to be more compassionate towards those who die by suicide and especially towards family and friends who are left bewildered by the act.

Religion seems to play some role in suicide prevention. The evidence is not strong and tends to be anecdotal but it seems that suicide is highest in Protestants, then next highest in Roman Catholics and those in the Jewish faith have a lower suicide rate than Roman Catholics. So how can religion help in reducing suicide? Again there is very little, if any, academic research to support current beliefs (Maris, Berman and Silverman, 2000). However, one early group of researchers noted that the suicide rate cross-matched with religion was higher in the Australian population than in similar religious groups in Ireland, England and Scotland (Burvill et al., 1983). However, when they compared the Australian suicide rates with the suicide rates in Irish, Scottish, and English emigrants to Australia they found little difference between them. Thus, they concluded that while a person was in their own country and practising their religious beliefs, there was a high possibility that in some way the person's religious belief system protected them.

For instance, hopelessness or despair about the future is highly correlated with suicide and religious belief offers hope for the future. In addition, the activities within a church such as attending services and meeting other people can give rise to an increased social network and support system, which in turn can buffer life's stresses.

However, one must bear in mind that much has changed in Britain and in Ireland in the last 20+ years. It could be that in current times religion may be a less protective factor than it used to be. Do people currently find solace in their religious beliefs? If so, then surely this belief could be tapped into in order to help prevent suicide? As religion is thought to be important to a large number of people, it would seem that research is very much needed in the area.

Attitudes to suicide-related behaviour

Discussion point: Spend a few moments to think about your attitude towards people who (1) think about suicide; (2) harm themselves; (3) try to kill themselves. Write down a few notes and revisit them after reading this chapter.

It has long been known that attitudes are a central tenet in the prediction of behavioural intentions and behaviour (Ajzen, 1985). If this is so, then the study of attitudes to suicide-related behaviour will be important to health caring professionals. For example, the core principles in psychotherapy, namely empathy, genuineness and acceptance (Rogers, 1961) are associated with positive client outcomes (Truax and Mitchell, 1971; Altschul, 1972), and they also reflect positive attitudes towards the person in need of therapeutic interaction (Rogers, 1975). Therefore, it could be assumed for example that negative attitudes in those who provide care or therapy would be likely to reduce the quantity and effectiveness of care given (Friedman *et al.*, 2006). Similarly, the attitudes of significant others may determine how they will respond to any form of suicide-related behaviour. For these reasons the study of attitudes to suicide-related behaviour in practitioners and even in significant others would be important.

Negative attitudes to suicide-related behaviour have existed in society for many years. As previously mentioned these attitudes were upheld by both legislation and religious doctrines. Within a hospital environment persons requiring care are subdivided by diagnoses. However, diagnoses can lead to dysfunctional attitudes by the staff towards persons who are so labelled. For instance, people who have taken an overdose frequently arrive in casualty in the early hours of the morning. More often than not they will smell of alcohol and this can create negative attitudes to such patients (Patel, 1975). Also, it has the potential for doctors and nurses to stereotype such persons (Muller and Poggenpoel, 1996). Stereotyping is an attempt to force people into certain categories or pigeonholes without considering unique circumstances or individual differences (Pennington, 1986). For example, 'overdoses are always drunk' and 'parasuicides don't really try to kill themselves' are negative forms of stereotyping. Sometimes staff rationalize that people admitted following a suicide-related behaviour are attention seeking, manipulative or that they cannot be helped (Vivekananda, 2000). Although stereotyping is not necessarily always negative (Leyens and Codol, 1988), it is rarely positive towards people who present in hospital following any form of suicide-related behaviour. The quality of the assessment will probably suffer if the patient is regarded as 'manipulative' or 'just another overdose' (Hawton and Catalan, 1987; Gibbs, 1990). Also, in the general hospital setting, it has been suggested that labelling patients as difficult can have a negative influence on the quality of care (Bentley, 1988; Carveth, 1995).

Negative attitudes to persons who exhibit suicide-related behaviour have been reported by UK researchers (Patel, 1975; Ramon, Bancroft and Skrimshire, 1975; Platt and Salter, 1987; Sidley and Renton, 1996) and elsewhere (Goldney and Bottrill, 1980; Pallikkathayil and Morgan, 1988; Bailey, 1994). Other researchers found that nurses display generally professional attitudes to persons admitted following some form of suicide-related behaviour, but appear to show negative personal attitudes after caring for them (Sidley and Renton, 1996). Nonetheless, the most commonly cited reactions include anger, frustration, lack of empathy, fear of involvement (Osborne, 1989), helplessness and even rage (Johnstone, 1997). In more recent times, Anderson (1997) reports on the frustration that accident and emergency nursing and medical staff feel when caring for people admitted following suicide-related behaviour. The end result of these emotions and fears can be avoidance behaviour (Osborne, 1989; Vivekananda, 2000) and a fear of saying the wrong thing (Bailey, 1994). Similarly, McLaughlin (1995) found that casualty nurses felt less competent in communicating with persons admitted following an overdose than with persons admitted with physical problems. There are possible links between these latter researchers' findings and Bandura's (1982) self-efficacy theory. It may be that some practitioners avoid such persons because they have difficulty communicating with them. For example, in one study where negative attitudes were reported, 83% of nurses felt that they would benefit from suicide-related education (Bailey, 1994). Furthermore, Friedman et al. (2006) concluded that there was a need for greater staff training in suicide-related behaviour in accident and emergency facilities.

Some very early research found that medical personnel such as physicians and junior doctors tended to place suicide-related behaviour in two categories: (1) those who really tried to end their lives, and (2) those that used suicide-related behaviour to manipulate others. Physicians, psychiatrists and nurses tended to have more sympathetic attitudes towards those who they thought of as having tried to kill themselves. However, they had more negative attitudes towards those who were deemed as not trying to kill themselves (Patel, 1975; Ramon, Bancroft and Skrimshire, 1975; Platt and Salter, 1987). In addition to that, psychiatrists tended to show more sympathetic attitudes and had a greater willingness to help such people than did medical doctors (Hawton, Marsack and Fagg, 1981; Platt and Salter, 1987). In other studies most staff felt that people admitted following a suicide-related behaviour should be cared for in a specialized unit rather than a general hospital setting (O'Brien and Stoll, 1977; Platt and Salter, 1987; Friedman *et al.*, 2006). However, there were no attitudinal differences between staff in a general hospital and staff in a specialist unit (Platt and Salter, 1987). A problem with this research was that participants in both facilities had completed similar training programmes.

Most of those persons who come into contact with the statutory services after a suicide-related behaviour will do so through the casualty department. Frequently such admissions will create high emotions and negative attitudes in staff. For example, a study carried out by McLaughlin (1994) reported that 80% of older casualty staff and 78% of younger casualty staff admitted hearing other staff say about an overdose patient, on more than one occasion, 'Why does he never do it right and save us a lot of trouble?' In addition, McLaughlin (1994), Anderson (1997) and McCann *et al.* (2006) reported that the more experienced casualty staff expressed more positive attitudes. However, in contrast, Friedman *et al.* (2006) found unhelpful attitudes among more experienced staff who had limited previous training in self-harm. In addition, Mackay and Barrowclough (2005) found that male staff and medical staff had more negative attitudes towards persons who self-harm. In contrast to other similar research, they also reported that medical staff saw less need for further training.

The study of mental health nurses' attitudes to suicidal behaviour in the UK, as elsewhere, is rare. What little empirical evidence exists suggests that mental health nurses have positive attitudes towards those admitted following suicide-related behaviour (Long and Reid, 1996; Anderson, 1997). While Long and Reid (1996) reported attitudes from mental health nurses in an acute setting, Anderson (1997) compared Community Mental Health Nurses' (CMHNs') attitudes to suicidal behaviour with those of casualty nurses. There are several points worth noting from these studies.

First, Anderson (1997) agreed with McLaughlin (1994) that more experienced casualty nurses have more positive attitudes to suicide-related behaviour than less experienced nurses. In contrast to this finding, Anderson (1997) reported that the less experienced CMHNs' attitudes to suicide-related behaviour are significantly more positive than the more experienced CMHNs. One would have assumed the reverse but there was no clear explanation for this finding. However, Anderson (1997) suggested that staffs' educational and practical experiences may have a hidden and complex influence on their attitudes.

Second, as Long and Reid (1996) report positive attitudes to suicide-related behaviour from only one acute setting, the results cannot be generalized to Northern Ireland as a whole or to the mental health nursing profession in general. In another study, McLaughlin (1997a) found that in general mental health nurses' attitudes to suicide-related behaviour were positive. McLaughlin (1997a) used four case vignettes in his questionnaire and each of these represented persons who (1) thought about suicide, (2) self-harmed, (3) had repeated admission and (4) attempted suicide. He also reported that while attitudes were very positive towards those who attempted suicide; their attitudes were less positive to those who self-harmed. In addition, Long and Reid (1996) reported that some mental health nurses found working with suicidal patients distressing and that they required additional education. It is worth noting that a number of authors have reported the need for further education and training in caring for and communicating with those admitted following suicide-related behaviour (Bailey, 1994; McLaughlin, 1995, 1997a; Anderson *et al.*, 2003; Crawford *et al.*, 2003; McCann *et al.*, 2006; Friedman *et al.*, 2006).

Attitudes of 'others' to suicidal behaviour

In a very early research project, Hawton, Bancroft and Simkin (1978) surveyed 40 patients classed as mentally ill and 40 patients admitted following an overdose. They found that both groups thought that overdoses reflected mental illness and that the behaviour was a reaction to life events. The overdose patients perceived the behaviour as being due to a disturbed state of mind. Also, more 'non-overdose' patients admitted that 'normal' people could take overdoses in difficult circumstances (Hawton, Bancroft and Simkin, 1978). In addition, James and Hawton (1985), in a survey of overdose patients' significant others, found that 41% of patients claimed to have suicidal ideation, while only 1% of their significant others (family) agreed. The significant others were more likely to attribute the behaviour to manipulative intentions. Nevertheless, both groups of participants agreed that overdosing was a means of alleviating distress.

Sometimes people who attend casualty do not wait for treatment and if seen they do not get followed up (Dennis, Owens and Jones, 1990). There is the possibility that having an unpleasant experience in casualty can be traumatic for the person who self-harms. For instance, Arnold (1994) found that when asked about the care they received, 69% of women were dissatisfied with the emergency services and some 96% of women were dissatisfied with mental health services. In addition, some authors found that those who self-harm are often ignored in casualty, they sometimes receive treatment without anaesthetic and have judgemental comments passed about them (Barstow, 1995; Pembroke and Smith, 1998). Similarly, Hemmings (1999) reported that patients felt that staff were judging and also punishing them for their self-harming behaviour. It is quite possible that some people who self-harm do not attend follow-up because of the way they are treated in hospital.

According to Ginn, Range and Hailey (1988) the community attitude is to ignore the suicidal behaviour. It is felt that suicidal behaviour is a private matter for the family and should not be made public knowledge. These authors feel that there is a need for community awareness and that the impact of suicidal behaviour on the community should be a matter for public debate. Finally, Morgan *et al.* (1996) surveyed eight groups of practitioners and compared their pre-lecture attitudes to suicide prevention with their post-lecture attitudes. Initially, they reported that up to one-third of the responses on the 10-question schedule were negative towards the concept of suicide prevention. However, there was a significant reduction in negative attitudes immediately after the lectures. They concluded that educational input of this kind should be regarded as an important element in the prevention of suicide.

Competency in interpersonal skills

Discussion point: For a few moments think about how competent you feel in communicating with people who (1) express thoughts about suicide, (2) try to kill themselves, or (3) self-harm.

The study of practitioners' attitudes to suicide-related behaviour has made the caring professions aware that negative attitudes to suicide-related behaviour do exist. There is no doubt about the existence of these negative attitudes as they are reported on time and time again. However, it is possible that other factors, different to attitudes, may impinge on the quantity and quality of care and produce either a reduction in empathetic listening or avoidance behaviour. For example, where it is observed that a practitioner exhibits limited communications with a person admitted following suicide-related behaviour in comparison to other patients, it may be inferred that the practitioner is avoiding that particular patient. This could be interpreted as an unfavourable attitude. In contrast, a questionnaire may show that the same practitioner has favourable attitudes towards suicidal patients. In the study of attitudes, this type of finding would not be novel. For example, in the classic study by La Piere (1934), attitudes may appear very positive on paper but on observation they may appear very different. This can also occur in hospital settings when it seems that some staff ignore or appear cold and impersonal towards persons who are admitted following suicide-related behaviour. The question that comes to mind is 'Do they really have a negative attitude towards the person?' A brief answer is – yes that might well be the case.

However, it might also be that some practitioners have difficulty, for whatever reason, in communicating with persons admitted following suicide-related behaviour. For example, this whole chapter deals with difficult areas that evoke strong emotions in people and that challenge practitioners' moral beliefs. Also, suicide-related behaviour is very contradictory in nature. Some practitioners can have difficulty in dealing with issues of that nature. It could be that these issues challenge their own professional, moral and religious belief systems.

However, if previous researchers' work (Ajzen, 1985; Bandura, 1982; Bailey, 1994; McLaughlin, 1995, 1997a) is considered, it may well be that nurses may, as suggested by Kalisch (1973), lack competence in the application of their communicating skills. For instance, McAllister *et al.* (2002) reported that staff felt helpless in dealing with the problems of those who self-harmed. In addition, McAllister *et al.* (2002) highlight the possibility that such helplessness in staff could be traumatizing for them. It is worth noting that for a long period of time, quite a number of authors have recommended an increase in staff training in caring for persons admitted following suicide-related behaviour (Bailey, 1994; McLaughlin, 1995, 1997a; McAllister *et al.*, 2002; Anderson *et al.*, 2003; Crawford *et al.*, 2003; McCann *et al.*, 2006; Friedman *et al.*, 2006). Thus, it is possible that lack of competence, in communicating, rather than unfavourable attitudes, may be the cause of avoidance behaviour in some practitioners.

From a different point of view, Nievaard (1987) found a clear link between the extent to which nurses experienced problems with physicians and management and the extent to which they had negative attitudes to patients. This type of frustration and interpersonal conflict within a health care team has the potential for what is termed as 'problem shifting'. Put simply, when management or other professionals pressurize practitioners, there is the potential for these staff to take out their frustration on patients. The question arises whether practitioners 'avoid' these clients as a result of negative attitudes towards them, or as a result of other factors within the working environment.

There is an assumption that educating staff about suicide-related behaviour could result in attitude change. In support of this, Morgan *et al.* (1996) found that negative attitudes towards the feasibility of suicide prevention in clinical practice can be reduced by a lecture. Similarly, McLaughlin (1997b) found that attitudes towards the treatment of mentally ill patients changed significantly as a result of lectures, and that this change remained significant following contact with mentally ill patients. These findings suggest that classroom teaching influences attitudes. Therefore, specific education on suicide-related behaviour and practice in interpersonal skills, as suggested by a number of authors, may lead to more positive attitudes and potentially more effective care for such persons.

Summary

This chapter focused on several contemporary issues that are associated with suicide-related behaviour. The concept of suicide-related behaviour and suicide in particular is very contradictory in its nature and its implementation. While some might see suicide as a selfish act that solves the person's difficulties, one has to ask: what about those who are left behind? Also, suicide and other forms of suicide-related behaviour are usually done alone and in private. Suicide-related behaviour challenges the person's religious beliefs and the beliefs of others. However, it seems that suicide is sometimes acceptable in some instances. For example, it is sometimes acceptable in times of war or when the person is experiencing insufferable pain from a terminal illness such as cancer.

Issues surrounding euthanasia and physician-assisted suicide have also been discussed. Is suicide ever rational? Is suicide ever right? The importance of these questions has been mooted and both of these questions have been addressed. However, while examples have been used to stimulate discussion, definitive answers have not been given here. It is expected that you will develop your own form of moral reasoning that will be influenced by your life's experiences and then moulded by your professional knowledge.

Attitudes to suicide-related behaviour have also been discussed. It is well known that some practitioners exhibit negative attitudes towards clients who are admitted following suicide-related behaviour. The strongest of these attitudes seem to be reserved for those people who self-harm. For example, there is some evidence that clients are ignored by some practitioners, are treated unfairly and have unpleasant comments expressed about them. There is a need to address these negative attitudes and a number of authors have called for this. However, this chapter also points out that there are other issues, different to attitudes that may also hinder the relationship between staff and patients. Some discussion is offered on these and recommendations are made.

Clarifying the terminology

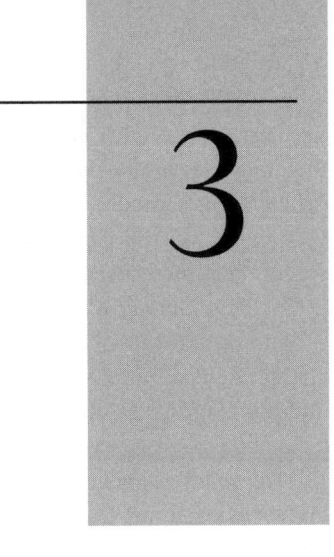

In Chapter 3 the following issues are explored:

1. The problem with too many different terms
2. Suicide intent
3. Lethality of method
4. Ambivalence
5. Risk-taking behaviour
6. The concept of suicide-related behaviour
7. Death-orientated suicide-related behaviour
8. Life-orientated suicide-related behaviour

The problem with too many different terms

There are numerous terms that are used to explain what suicide-related behaviour is. However, just because a practitioner can put a name to a particular behaviour, does not mean that they can understand it. From the outset, it is important to acknowledge that most, if not all, terms used were meant well and make points that are well taken and seem justifiable when originally proposed. However, in more recent times while some terms may cause ambiguity or interpretation difficulties between multidisciplinary team members, some other terms could be seen as being downright derogatory towards a person in crisis and in deep despair. It is therefore incumbent on all practitioners to ensure that the terms used in their speciality areas are clear, unambiguous and do not offend the person to whom they are applied. Ever since Durkheim (1897/1951) defined suicide the debate for a common set of terms or nomenclature has been ongoing. While O'Carroll *et al.* (1996) proposed a common nomenclature; it seems that in more recent times there is still difficulty in gaining global agreement (Silverman, 2005, 2006). This chapter will highlight the debate on terminology that is frequently used to explain the phenomenon of suicide-related behaviour. In addition, this chapter will summarize the main components within suicide-related behaviour and it will present a diagram that explains the pathways within suicide-related behaviour.

The work of mental health professionals focuses on an abstract concept known as the mind. Even since the great debate between Watson and McDougall (1929), the concept of the mind has continued to generate much debate especially among social scientists and psychologists. In brief, there is an assumption that people think and then act accordingly. The primary assumption is that the thinking component relates to the activity within a person's mind. The person may think about or consider a matter and then instigate a course of action or behaviour as a result of their thoughts. From an observant point of view, the behaviour will be observable and more often than not it will be measurable. Put very simply, practitioners can observe the behaviour of a person and then verbally report on that behaviour. Unfortunately, the same cannot be said about a person's thought processes. For example, practitioners can see a person's behaviour and can then subjectively infer what the person was thinking at the time of the behaviour. That does not mean that the practitioner's inference is correct. Similarly, the personal issues that people present with can be subjective in nature. Practitioners may have difficulty in explaining these issues and sometimes ambiguity is an all too frequent problem.

In suicide-related behaviour, the terminology used by practitioners tries to focus on the person's behaviour (self-injury, self-poisoning, parasuicide) or on the practitioner's understanding of the person's intention (gestured suicide, attention-seeking). Sometimes the terms used are open to misinterpretation by other professionals. Currently there are quite a number of different terms being used that try to describe the phenomenon of suicide-related behaviour. On occasions the interpretation of many of these terms has the potential to create confusion in practitioners. It is not that practitioners are themselves confused but that the terms being used by them are either ambiguous or misunderstood. For example, until recently I was very much in agreement with the term 'parasuicide' as proposed by Kreitman *et al.* (1969) and discussed in Kreitman (1977). In parasuicide, there is no intention to die. However, in more recent times I have heard some colleagues suggest that in parasuicide there is low suicide intent. For me, that suggests a degree of confusion. For instance, how can some professionals, including myself, think that in parasuicide there is no intention to kill oneself while other professionals think that there is some (low) intention to kill oneself? Put it another way, if a practitioner suspects that a person intends to kill themself or a person expresses an intention to kill themself, does it matter whether the intent is high or low? Sometimes, individual practitioners may use different terms to describe the same behaviour. On a number of occasions I have heard professional colleagues including practitioners debate, discuss and strongly disagree with each other over what particular terms mean and how terms should be used. On some occasions I found that the professional who was perceived as being the most senior in the team usually won the debate and their choice of term was that which was used by the rest of the team. In doing so most of the team, if not all, used the same terminology. This type of local conformity brings some consensus of agreement to the team. A local agreement is one thing but gaining a national or a global agreement seems to be more difficult (Silverman, 2005, 2006).

At a national level, there are many differently qualified mental health practitioners who work with people with histories of suicide-related behaviour. Some of these practitioners are employed in teams in government statutory health boards. However, other professionals work in the voluntary non-statutory sector. In addition, an increasing number of mental health practitioners are beginning to work in the private sector. Many of these practitioners will use their own terminology to describe the type of suicide-related behaviour exhibited by persons who are referred to them for therapy. The difficulties arise here because different professionals will more than likely use different terminology. Also, information is not termed or coded in an agreed unified way by different teams or facilities. In effect, the absence of such agreements means that it would be less than useless in trying to compare data from these statutory, non-statutory and private facilities. In addition, if these difficulties exist at local and at national level, what about a global agreement? In considering the terms used in suicide-related behaviour, how would you or your health care team members interpret the following real case scenario?

Case vignette 15

Jane Brown is an 18-year-old Information Technology student who lives with her parents in a quiet suburban area. She gets on well with her father and can confide in him. However, she does not get on with her mother. In recent times there have been frequent arguments between Jane and her mother and she finds that she cannot confide in her mother. Also, in the past few months Jane has wanted to get away from home and to become more independent in life.

She has been going steady with her boyfriend Ron for almost a year and she has hoped that they will get married. Recently, however, things have not been going well with her and Ron. In the last month she and Ron have had a number of serious arguments and Jane thinks that Ron is less interested in her now. On the night before her admission to hospital they went to a party together. Soon after arriving at the party Ron more or less ignored her and spent most of the evening dancing with other girls. Jane became very upset and left on her own. She walked around the town for some time before returning home. When she got home, her mother came out of her room and criticized her for being so late and asked where she'd been. Jane started to argue, but then quickly went into the bathroom and swallowed 10 paracetamol tablets. Her father came into the bathroom and found out what had happened, and took her immediately to the accident and emergency department of the local hospital. While in hospital, a nurse asked her why she did it and she replied that she just wanted to sleep. Also, she had a gastric lavage to remove the remains of the tablets and was advised by the Senior House Officer to remain in hospital overnight for observation.

On the following day her medical charts noted the following reports:

(a) Senior House Officer: Patient admitted to A&E at 3.30 a.m. after deliberately self-harming herself by ingesting 10 paracetamol. Gastric lavage administered and stomach contents emptied. Remains of 10 tablets recovered. Advised to remain overnight for observation and assessment. To be seen by Psychiatric Liaison Nurse and possible transfer to Medical Ward.

(b) Psychiatric Liaison Nurse: Patient admitted to A&E at 3.30 a.m. after attempted suicide by overdose (10 x paracetamol swallowed). Following stabilization by A&E team, she was transferred to Medical Ward. She was emotionally upset because she and her boyfriend had fallen out. However, she has agreed to see the counselling therapist in the morning.

(c) House Officer on Medical Ward: Patient transferred from A&E at 5 a.m. to Medical Ward following a manipulative self-harm gesture by deliberately ingesting 10 paracetamol tablets. Bloods have been sent to the laboratory. Vital signs to be observed every 30 minutes. To be seen by the psychiatric counsellor in the morning.

When the counselling therapist arrives to see Jane (s)he has very little information to go on. There are three different diagnostic terms used in each report (deliberate self-harm, suicide attempt, and manipulative self-harm gesture). In this case the counselling therapist is unsure whether or not Jane has tried to kill herself. In order to find out what really happened the counselling therapist has to start from the beginning to build a picture of why Jane swallowed 10 paracetamol in the early hours of the morning. In the time before the arrival of the counselling therapist, a number of health care staff will have already seen the reports and have made their own judgements on Jane's care needs.

Discussion point: In a small group (no more than six students) spend 10–15 minutes discussing your answer to the following question and make sure that you include rationale for your decisions: if you were the counselling therapist what would be your interpretation of Jane's behaviour? Write down some notes on your decisions and compare these notes with other groups.

The above scenario is not uncommon and the problem of ambiguity in the terms used in suicide-related behaviour is not new. Since Durkheim's (1897/1951) influential work and particularly since its translation into English there has been a consistent effort to clarify and simplify the increasing number of different terms that were being used. For example, classification schemes have been proposed by Schmidt, O'Neal and Robins (1954), Shneidman (1968), Pokorny (1974), Ellis (1988), van Egmond and Diekstra (1990). In addition, Arensman and Kerkhof (1996) and Wagner, Wong and Jobes (2002) have added considerably to the debate. Also, the weight of important research-based bodies such as the World Health Organization (Schmidtke *et al.*, 1996) and the American Association of Suicidology (O'Carroll *et al.*, 1996; Silverman, 2005, 2006), who have sincere interests in the reduction of global suicide-related behaviour, have added to the discussion. In addition, in Ireland there is the Irish Association of Suicidology, the National Suicide Research Foundation and the National Parasuicide Registry. In Great Britain there is the Centre for Suicide Research in Oxford. These are only a few examples of excellent bodies, which have the power to draw together terminology that is commonly understood. These bodies have a wealth of professionals who have vested interests in the reduction of suicide-related behaviour and who are more than capable of producing unambiguous terminology in suicide-related behaviour for use by practitioners from all caring professions. Unfortunately, it seems that in over 50 years none of these past efforts at clarification has been adopted on a national or global basis. While Silverman (2005) points out the difficulties in obtaining global agreement on a common set of terms, it still seems strange that given the importance of the topic a common set of terms has not been agreed. However, recently Silverman (2006) has called for an international summit to discuss the terminology used in suicide-related behaviour.

Furthermore, while statutory bodies are well recognized for the work they do, it must be acknowledged that there are numerous non-statutory and charitable organizations operating in Ireland, Great Britain and indeed further afield. Many of these organizations are usually highly focused on the people they care for. Many will provide assessment, caring and other therapeutic responses for people experiencing psychache including people with histories of suicide-related behaviour. Many readers will immediately think of the Samaritans as a major charitable organization that provides a much needed and worthwhile service. However, in my own geographical area and in addition to the Samaritans there are two other organizations providing services for people with histories of suicide-related behaviour. Specifically, these are: (1) zest – healing the hurt and (ii) LATCH (Listening and Talking Can Help). In addition to these there are a number of practitioners providing private counselling practices. Organizations such as these have a lot to offer regarding the type of care required and in particular the terminology used by practitioners in suicide-related behaviour.

To make a point it might be a useful exercise to personalize what is meant by terminology. For instance, we all like to be called by our proper names and on some occasions by our proper titles. How do we feel when someone replaces our name by a nickname? Some may say that they feel all right about it. However, that may be so depending on who is calling who by what nickname. Pet names or nicknames may have a place in close family circles and in loving relationships. However, both pet names and nicknames do not have a place in the professional world. For example, nicknames can be derogatory; they can also be used to exert control over another human being; and to make vulnerable people feel small or inadequate. In this way, the use of nicknames can be viewed as a form of verbal abuse and bullying. In addition, a nickname can create negative attitudes by others towards the person. Similarly, the use of some terms can appear derogatory and can create negative attitudes in practitioners towards persons whom they choose to label. As practitioners communicate both verbally and by writing in a person's case notes they need to be careful that the terms they use are not derogatory towards their persons. For example, what would Jane think if she knew that someone wrote in her case notes that her action was described by a practitioner as manipulative? Was Jane suicidal? If she was not suicidal, why say that she attempted suicide. Also, as a practitioner reading these words and not having met Jane, what would you think about her? How would you interpret the term 'suicide gesture' or the term 'attempted suicide'?

From my own point of view I always believed in using terms that were, at least to me, unambiguous and easily understood by other persons. Sadly, in suicide-related behaviour the terminology that is used is not always clear. Nonetheless, the terms used by all practitioners in suicide-related behaviour should accurately focus on and categorize the person's intention at the time of the behaviour. Unfortunately, when it comes to suicide-related behaviour, estimating someone's intentions is easier said than done. It is well known that a person's intention at the time of the suicide-related behaviour and the seriousness (potential lethality) of the behaviour are the two main constructs that define all forms of suicide-related behaviour. Therefore, any useful definition should recognize these constructs in some form or other. Prior to exploring some specific and potentially useful terms it might be worthwhile mentioning some of the terms that have been previously used to define the phenomenon of suicide. These are listed, in no particular order of importance, in Boxes 3.1–3.3.

In Box 3.1, a number of terms that seek to define whether or not a person is thinking about the possibility of suicide are mentioned. A key question here is whether or not each of the terms means the same thing to different professionals.

Box 3.1 Terms used to define a person's thoughts about suicide.

Suicide-related ideation*	Suicide threat	Suicidal intention
Suicidal motivation	Suicidal expression	Suicidal thoughts
Considering suicide	Suicidal ideation	Morbid ruminations

* Main focus in this book

For example, when a person threatens suicide, does that mean that he or she is thinking about suicide?

Discussion point: In a small group (no more than six students) spend 10–15 minutes discussing the following scenario: if a person says to you, 'I feel that life is not worth living any more', what would you think? Which term in Box 3.1 would you use? Why would you use that term in favour over another term? Also, how would you report or record it in the person's notes?

In Box 3.2 there are quite a number of terms that I am aware of that have been used to specify a person's behaviour prior to their admission to hospital. It

Box 3.2 Terms used to define behaviour related to suicide.

Attempted suicide*	Pseudosuicide	Non-completed suicide
Non-fatal suicide	Parasuicide	Gestured suicide
Instrumental behaviour	Self-injury	Self-harm*
Self-abuse	Self-harm behaviour	Self-destructive behaviour
Self-injurious behaviour	Self-inflicted injury	Self-directed violence
Self-mutilation	Self-suffocation	Self-strangulation
Self-poisoning	Deliberate self-injury	Deliberate self-harm
Intentional self-injury	Intentional self-harm	Intentional injury
Suicide gesture	Self-wounding	Self-cutting
Wrist slashing	Symbolic wounding	Suicide-related behaviour*
Cosmic roulette	Repeaters	Malingering
Autoaggression	Attention-seeking	Indirect self-destructive behaviour
Burners	Overdose	Suicidal behaviour
Trauma re-enactment syndrome		Instrumental suicide-related behaviour

* Main focus in this book

Box 3.3	Terms used to define suicide.	
Suicide*	Self-death	Self-destruction
Self-induced annihilation	Self-induced death	Deliberate death
Completed suicide	Self-inflicted death	Self-murder
Direct self-destruction	Focal suicide	Intentional suicide

* Main focus in this book

is possible that there are more terms than I am unaware of. However, the above list of terms serves the purpose of identifying where ambiguity and confusion can begin. There are arguments to say that injury is different to poisoning and that the behaviour itself is important. There are also arguments to say that some behaviour is potentially more lethal than others.

Discussion point: In a small group (no more than six students) spend 10–15 minutes discussing the following scenario. Suppose there were two persons on your ward who were admitted following non-accidental trauma. Let us say that one person had taken an overdose of paracetamol and the other person had shot him or herself. Which of the terms in Box 3.2 would you use to define the behaviours of each of the persons? Secondly, what rationale would you give for your use of those terms?

In Box 3.3, a number of terms that seek to define how a person killed themselves are mentioned. A key question here is whether or not each of the terms means the same thing to different professionals.

Discussion point: In a small group (no more than six students) spend 10–15 minutes discussing the following scenario: if you heard that a person had killed themselves, what terms in Box 3.3 would you use and why?

In this book the main focus will be on the exploration of the terms in Boxes 3.1–3.3 that are indicated with an asterisk (*). Most, if not all, of the above terms have a theoretical basis that reflects the position of the author(s) that proposed them. While each of the terms in Boxes 3.1–3.3 above contain both flaws and fair comment, even a brief exploration of the relevant literature will reveal that there is some confusion in what each of the terms mean and indeed there are inconsistencies among practitioners in how each term is interpreted. This can create difficulties for mental health practitioners, particularly when they are keeping abreast of the literature pertaining to suicide-related behaviour. For example, it is common to find in mental health research reports terms such as parasuicide, attempted suicide, overdose and deliberate self-harm all being used to describe the same behaviour regardless of the person's intentions. Also, in some books and even in some research-based scripts it is not uncommon to find different terms being used alternatively on the same page to describe the same behaviour.

In some research studies of people who have been admitted to hospital following an overdose, it seems that all cases of overdose are included irrespective of the person's intentions. To ensure clarity it would be very helpful if such studies included separate tables that correspond with: (1) persons who intended killing themselves, and (2) persons who had no intention of killing themselves. Other than having overdose as a common denominator, many readers would find it difficult to interpret any additional findings in such research reports and compare them with data in other research reports. Many research studies are well conceived and conducted by well-meaning researchers. Unfortunately, in many cases, because of ambiguity in the terminology and in the definitions used, the data is not directly comparable with similar research reported elsewhere. If terms such as parasuicide, deliberate self-harm, intentional self-harm, self-destructive behaviour, and self-injurious behaviour are all defined in a similar way or are perceived by practitioners as being the same as self-harm, then why not strive to use one agreed term?

In addition to the above, one of the difficulties with too many terms is that somewhere along the road, some terms become associated with negative attitudes. For instance, the term 'commit suicide' is used very frequently and would seem to be inoffensive. However, the word 'commit' is also frequently linked with criminal activity as in 'commit a crime'. For this reason relatives of those who have died by suicide have objected to the word 'commit' being used to describe a suicide. In addition, it has been recommended that the word 'commit' is no longer used in relation to suicide (NICE, 2004a). Furthermore, McLaughlin (1997a) found that practitioners had less positive attitudes and lower intentions to communicate with a person whose action was perceived as self-harm than they were with a person whom they considered to have attempted suicide. Differences here seemed to revolve around the practitioner's opinion as to whether the person 'genuinely tried to kill him or herself'. In recent times, the use of the terms 'deliberate' and 'intentional' in relation to self-harm have been criticized and it has been recommended that practitioners no longer use the terms (NICE, 2004a). Previously, Barker (2003) had criticized the use of the word 'deliberate' being linked to self-harm or self-injury as it had created an image of blaming the person for the act. For example, the term gives the impression that practitioners are saying to a person 'you deliberately did that'. Of course the person did it. The person may have done it impulsively, deliberately, and intentionally or (s)he may even have planned to do it for a lengthy period of time.

A similar argument can be put forward for the term 'suicide threat'. Sometimes, the person is informing family, friends or practitioners of the possibility that they might harm themselves rather than 'threatening' others that they are going to harm themselves. It is not for the practitioner to apportion blame, unintentionally or not, but to find out why the person carried out the behaviour or says that they are going to do it. It is not that any of the terms in Boxes 3.1–3.3 are wrong. In fact most if not all the terms have stemmed from well-meaning concepts and from well-meaning authors and practitioners who have attempted to describe the specific behaviour in a clear and unambiguous way. Unfortunately, by increasing the number of terms from which practitioners can choose, these attempts to describe a person's suicide-related behaviour have only added to the confusion.

If practitioners are expected to carry out accurate risk assessments, provide appropriate psychological care, and share professional knowledge and research findings then it is important that they use the same terminology and the same definitions. This has implications both nationally and globally. Unfortunately, national and global agreements on terminology and definitions are nonexistent. In the absence of an agreed terminology, mental health practitioners may take the chance that their decisions, based on their own standards or criteria, are correct. Such decisions could be well made but they may also be wide of the mark. In clinical decisions, especially in the assessment of a person's care needs and in recommending and implementing caring responses, the lack of uniformity among practitioners runs the risk of:

1. misinterpreting the person's behaviour;
2. conveying different interpretations to other professional colleagues;
3. restricting the use of potential therapeutic interventions;
4. being inconsistent in the type of therapeutic interventions offered;
5. limiting follow-up care;
6. offering no uniformity in recording and comparing data.

The lack of uniformity in terminology can lead to difficulties in any or all of the above six areas. At no time can practitioners – particularly in this current technologically advanced world – afford the mistake of having ambiguous terminology in its vocabulary. Currently, on the subject of suicidology and as illustrated in Boxes 3.1–3.3, there is much room for ambiguity and misunderstanding. While such a state exists then it will remain difficult to agree on therapeutic approaches to care and to compare data in research reports.

Suicide intent

In trying to understand why professionals are inconsistent in their interpretation of a person's suicide-related behaviour, it is useful to think about the two main constructs that currently underline and define all suicide-related behaviours. These constructs are: (1) the person's intention to die and (2) the lethality (seriousness) of the behaviour. It is worthwhile noting that for over 30 years the critical role played by the person's intention to die at the time of their behaviour has been recognized and acknowledged. In addition, authors still maintain its importance (O'Carroll *et al.*, 1996; Wagner, Wong and Jobes, 2002; Haw *et al.*, 2003; Silverman, 2005, 2006; Andriessen, 2006).

Discussion point: In a small group (no more than six students) spend 10–15 minutes discussing your experience of measuring a person's intention at the time of a suicide-related behaviour. Have you ever used scales to measure a person's intention? In your opinion how useful did you find these scales?

In exploring the concept of suicide intent, O'Carroll *et al.* (1996) made a very strong case for the need to have a unified nomenclature or a set of commonly understood and logically defined terms. Rudd (1997) and Dear (1997) gave very strong support to the proposed nomenclature. O'Carroll *et al.* (1996) suggested two broad categories which they called: (1) 'Instrumental Suicide-Related Behaviour' and (2) 'Suicidal Acts'. Each of these categories has at its core the person's intention or non-intention to kill him or herself at the time of the behaviour. For example, they suggested that there was a zero intention to die in the 'Instrumental Behaviour' category. However, in the 'Suicidal Acts' category the person at some non-zero level intended to die. Both these statements make it very clear that on one side there is no suicide intent while on the other there is suicide intent. Furthermore, Dear (1997) suggested some refinements to the nomenclature. For example, he felt that it was misleading to label suicide-related behaviours (where there is no intent to die) as 'instrumental' when suicidal acts (where there is intent to die) are every bit as instrumental (Dear, 1997, p. 409). From a definitional point of view all behaviours, with the exception of reflex behaviours, are instrumental in nature. However, Dear (1997) had difficulty in suggesting a different term that would avoid implying manipulation or minimizing the importance of the behaviour. In more recent times, Silverman (2005) has made it very clear that the term 'Instrumental Suicide-Related behaviour' is a 'no go'. This then leaves practitioners with the question: what do we call those behaviours that are non-accidentally self-inflicted and where it seems that the person had no intention to kill him or herself? It would seem that finding out the person's intention at the time of their behaviour would be the best and most promising starting point (Andriessen, 2006).

However, finding out about a person's intention is difficult and easier said than done. A practitioner can ask the person directly about their intentions at the time of the behaviour, but it is not unusual for a person to deny or minimize any suicidal intent. Conversely, a person could claim to have a high suicide intent when the opposite is true. In addition, the person may be ambivalent about their behaviour. Ambivalence is common in suicide-related behaviour (Shneidman, 1985) and it can make it difficult for practitioners to come to a conclusion regarding the person's intentions. If the practitioner relies only on the person's self-reported suicide intent, then their assessment could be erroneous. However, there are some tools that can help the practitioner in their assessment. For instance, the very early Suicide Intent Scale by Beck, Schuyler and Herman (1974) and the later Pierce's Intent Scale (Pierce, 1977) are as useful today as they have always been. From an anecdotal point of view, I have found that using these scales on their own can create false high scores; however, when combined with a full in-depth psychosocial assessment, these scales can give the astute practitioner a better than average chance of eliciting a person's intentions at the time of their suicide-related behaviour.

The importance of a person's intent at the time of their suicide-related behaviour should not be underestimated. At the time of someone's death, an autopsy of events may or may not reveal a suicide intention and any difficulty here must involve coroners in the deliberations. However, while accurately recording how people die is important, it is the viewpoint in this book that estimating the future risk of suicide in any individual is of the utmost importance. Indeed, Andriessen (2006) constructs a very valid argument and makes this point very clear. Certainly, the successful measurement of suicide intent in an individual is without doubt going to be the 'holy grail' of Suicidology in the future.

Lethality of method

The second construct that defines suicide-related behaviour is that of how lethal the behaviour is. One could easily assume that the lethality of any suicide-related behaviour would be objectively defined. This is true in some cases but not in all cases. For example, let's take a hypothetical case where a person has been shot in the head and survived. For the purpose of debate, let's say that while in hospital this person admitted that they had shot themself and had wanted to die. Most reasonable professionals would determine that the person has survived a very serious suicide attempt. Let us take another but contrasting scenario. Whereas deep cuts that sever major blood vessels are potentially fatal, superficial scratch marks to the skin are not fatal. Should a teenager with superficial scratch marks be admitted to hospital and while there admit no intention to die, then practitioners may rightly or wrongly judge that the person was not suicidal and that the behaviour was a form of suicide gesture/self-harm/parasuicide/deliberate self-harm or they may use some other such term. Generally speaking, when a case has a very high intention of suicide and a very lethal behaviour or when a case has no suicide intention and low lethal behaviour, then most practitioners can make fairly accurate judgements.

For instance, in a recent study, Wagner, Wong and Jobes (2002) investigated mental health professionals' interpretation of the term suicide attempt. Each participant was presented with 10 case studies. They found that when the behaviour was clearly very serious or non-serious both suicidologists and other mental health professionals were able to identify reliably whether the behaviour was an attempted suicide or not. However, both groups were less able to do so when the behaviour was less clear. For example, suppose a person was admitted to hospital following a self-inflicted gun shot wound to the head and this person was adamant that (s)he had no intention of killing themselves! What would any practitioner think? Or how would a practitioner react to a teenager who is admitted to hospital with superficial scratch marks to the wrist and expresses a wish to die? It is difficult for the practitioner to make clear judgements about these latter two cases. This is because the verbal responses contrast with the degree of lethality used in the behaviour. Which should the practitioner believe – the verbal response or the lethality of the behaviour?

In another example, some practitioners would consider taking an overdose as being non-serious suicide-related behaviour. The reason for this is that many people who take an overdose survive it. However, analysis of government annual statistics shows that quite a number of people in the United Kingdom do die as a result of overdosing. The availability of analgesics such as paracetamol has been cited as a main reason why some people choose to overdose (Hawton *et al.*, 2000). However, since 1998, legislation has been introduced in the United Kingdom to limit the pack size of some analgesics that are available over the counter (Hawton, 2002). Similar legislation was introduced in the Republic of Ireland in October 2001. Thus, while on the one hand taking an overdose can be quite serious and life-threatening, on the other hand, because there is a chance of survival, some practitioners may mistakenly perceive it as being of low lethality.

Judging the lethality of a suicide-related behaviour can be fraught with difficulty and should not be used alone as an indicator of suicide intent. It is very important that practitioners should also find out whether the person tried to kill him or herself. Wagner, Wong and Jobes (2002) make the point that while some professionals might weigh the person's intention more so than lethality, others may weight lethality more than intention. For me, on a very personal note, any activity that is perceived as lethal is lethal. There is no activity that is less lethal than another lethal method. Putting it very simply, each of hanging, cutting and taking an overdose are potentially lethal. Each of these methods frequently result in the suicidal death of people, therefore none is more or less lethal than the other. I therefore take the viewpoint that while the method a person chooses to kill themselves is important, it is less important than their intention to kill themselves. Nonetheless, all practitioners must weigh up the information that they are presented with, including lethality, in order to form an opinion about the person's suicide-related behaviour.

Ambivalence

In addition to suicide intent and the lethality of any particular behaviour, a person's thoughts about dying can be compounded by another type of thinking. Sometimes, it seems that these people do not care whether they live or die.

Discussion point: In a small group (no more than six students) spend 10–15 minutes discussing your experience of talking to a person who was admitted to your ward following a suicide-related behaviour and who seemed ambivalent about their behaviour and their care. Write down some notes from your group and compare these with notes from other groups.

Ambivalence is a common cognitive state in suicide-related behaviour (Shneidman, 1985). In being ambivalent the person experiences simultaneous contradictory feelings. For instance, Shneidman (1985) makes the point that in ambivalence a person is convinced that they have to kill themselves yet the person would also like to be helped. The subject of ambivalence is raised here as Dear (1997) highlighted a difference between an intention to die and a preparedness to die. For example, in the aftermath of a suicide-related behaviour some people will make it very clear that they had no intention of dying nor did they expect to die. However, others may state that at the time of the behaviour they did not care whether or not they died. This latter statement suggests that the person is ambivalent. For some practitioners, the state of ambivalence may be problematic. However, Dear (1997, p. 409) rightly makes the point that ambivalence suggests that the person is prepared to die and that this is above zero in terms of an intention to die. In other words ambivalence fits into O'Carroll *et al.*'s (1996) non-zero level. Therefore, any behaviour where the person is prepared to die or intended to die must be taken very seriously by practitioners.

At this point it would be useful to point out that Silverman (2005) criticized the term 'non-zero intent' (O'Carroll *et al.*, 1996) as being too broad and too vague. However, O'Carroll *et al.* (1996) make it very clear that there is a difference between absolutely no intent to kill oneself (zero intent) and any level, no matter how trivial or slight, of intent to kill oneself. They use the term non-zero, which means that the person has some intent. It may be low intent or slight intent but the fact remains that it is still intent. Similarly, in this book, the term non-zero is adopted and accepted for what O'Carroll *et al.* (1996) meant it to be. In effect, when this criterion is applied here, then being ambivalent about life and death means that the person has some suicidal intent.

The definitional differences between being prepared to die and having intended to die are acknowledged and do not need to be repeated in this book. In addition, the importance of a person's intention and their preparedness to die are also acknowledged. However, an overriding consideration in this book is that both are important and that both should be given equal measure and equal attention by practitioners. For example, if a person's help-seeking behaviour is not effectively responded to and their intention is to die, then there is a very high chance that the end result will be that the person will die. Similarly, there is also a very high chance that the ambivalent person will die if their help-seeking behaviour is not effectively responded to. Thus, it is asserted in this book that ambivalence is a very serious type of thinking in suicide-related behaviour. However, because a person is ambivalent does not mean that they are entirely orientated towards death. One positive point associated with ambivalence is that the person would also be willing to accept therapeutic help. In being ambivalent there is room for negotiation and there is the possibility of moving a person from a death-orientated position to a life-orientated position. This point will be further explored in Chapter 8 (Therapeutic responses to suicide-related behaviour).

Risk-taking behaviour

While some eminent authors distinguish between risk-taking thoughts and suicide-related thoughts (suicidal related ideation), others put risk-taking behaviour on a continuum, which has tattooing one's body at one extreme and suicide at other extreme. It is important to realize that all or most of us, at some time in our lives, have engaged in risk-taking behaviour to some degree or another. This does not mean that all of us are suicidal in nature. However, risk taking can be part and parcel of normal daily living. In fact it would be a very dull life if it were devoid of all risks. Through taking risks people can learn, develop and grow. Some very common examples, and also some illegal examples, of risk-taking behaviour include: smoking, crossing a busy road, recreational drug use, unprotected sexual activity, drinking alcohol, swimming, rugby, bungee jumping, rock-climbing, sky-diving, mountaineering and speeding while driving. In fact the list of risk-taking behaviours is almost endless and can include all types of both legal and illegal behaviours.

It is very obvious that some risk-taking behaviours are clearly sensation-seeking activities and participants derive a high level of excitement and pleasure from them. Certainly, Apter (1992) would agree with this. For instance, Apter (1992) argues that in order to experience high arousal and excitement, some people need to expose themselves to sufficient danger and yet feel protected through their own competence and skill. There is no doubt that in some of the activities mentioned above there is a very high level of danger. However, in most, if not all, such activities safety is paramount and it is the responsibility of each participant, the organizer or both parties. Thus, while there is inherent danger in risk-taking behaviour, this danger can be minimized through preparation, training, expertise and the use of safety equipment. For example, in extreme sports such as rock-climbing a lead climber who intends to climb a cliff will take precautions. For instance, (s)he will put on a harness; they will attach a rope to this harness and tie it on with a failsafe knot such as a figure of eight. On their way up the cliff (s)he will place their own protective equipment into cracks in the rock or place slings over rocky projections. This protective equipment is attached to a specialized piece of equipment called a 'karabiner'. The rope that the lead climber is attached to is passed through the karabiner and down to a second person (the belayer) who is also attached to the end of the rope and safely tied into the cliff. In the event of the leader taking a fall, the safety of the lead climber will be dependent on three things: (1) the protective equipment (s)he has used, (2) the quality or soundness of the rock and (3) the ability of the belayer in preventing him or her from falling. In some cases, such as in training courses protective equipment may have already been placed by others. Similarly, in bungee jumping safety equipment is placed by the participant or by the organizers. In addition, and in a completely different context, most, if not all, children are taught how to cross a busy road safely. With all of these activities there are inherent dangers. Yet in each of these risk-taking activities the danger is minimized by education, training, or by the competent skill of the person.

However, an astute observer will note that any person can also choose to take part in risk-taking behaviour without the use of safety or protective equipment. This then puts the risk-taking activity into a new dimension where the safety of the people is entirely dependent on their own ability to perform the activity competently. In effect, this is a demonstration of practical skill and competence in a dangerous activity where the risk of failure could result in either serious injury or even death. Nonetheless, it is acknowledged that a person's practical skill can ensure safety.

However, in contrast there are activities that are considered high risk and whose outcome does not depend on education, training or expertise. For example, Russian Roulette is frequently defined as a game. However, it is a deadly game where the chance of death is very high and where the person playing it challenges the probability that they might die. In effect, the person's life is entirely dependent on fate and no amount of preparation, training or skill can alter the outcome. Thus, Russian Roulette is very different from all other risk-taking behaviours. Indeed, Maris, Berman and Silverman (2000, p. 451) say that it is a gamble with death and that 'the spoils of victory are nothing more than what one began with – one's life'. While safety and competence frequently feature in many risk-taking activities, that is certainly not the case in Russian Roulette. Finally, when risk-taking behaviour ends in the death or serious injury of the person, it can be a very difficult area in inquests. For example, was the injury or death an accident or did the person knowingly put their life at risk with the intention of dying or being seriously injured?

It is acknowledged that people can die as a result of risk-taking behaviour. However, in this book, risk-taking thoughts or risk-taking behaviours are not viewed in the same light as suicide-related thoughts or suicide-related behaviour. While risk-taking thoughts or behaviours such as mountain climbing, skydiving, sexual promiscuity, smoking and other similar activities can result in death, injury or ill health, the person's intention at the time was not focused on them harming or killing themselves. Therefore, it is asserted in this book, that while risk-taking behaviour can result in ill health, injury, or death it is not related to a person's preparedness to die nor to any intention to harm him or herself or die at any given point. For example, risk-taking thoughts or behaviours can only be related when there is evidence that a person carried out a risk-taking behaviour such as climbing a mountain not caring whether they came back alive or dead or intending to die or harm themselves while climbing the mountain. Similarly, although Mann *et al.* (1999) found an association between smoking and suicide-related behaviour in psychiatric persons, many people smoke a cigarette because they enjoy it, not because they want to die from smoking. In many ways risk-taking behaviour is weighed up by the person in terms of their enjoyment of the activity, the adrenaline rush afterwards, the risk to themselves and their ability to accomplish the activity safely.

The concept of suicide-related behaviour

As stated earlier, the terminology used by practitioners is very important because these same practitioners need to ensure that they are talking the same language and have the same meaning. Since the 1950s there have been a number of authors who have tried to classify and clarify the terms used in suicide-related behaviour. Of these, the terminology suggested by O'Carroll *et al.* (1996) and the update by Silverman (2005, 2006) are very useful. Unfortunately, it seems that such efforts are having difficulty in being adopted on a global basis. This is disappointing and even more so when one considers the number of international bodies such as the World Health Organization and the American Association of Suicidology that have the power to produce terminology that is globally accepted by both persons and practitioners. Both Rudd (1997) and Dear (1997) were very strong in their support for the nomenclature proposed by O'Carroll *et al.* (1996) and I also concur with their comments. In common with Rudd (1997), I believe that with regard to suicide-related behaviour a universally accepted set of terminology is (1) essential if practitioners are to understand the phenomenon of suicide-related behaviour, (2) a foundation for clinical care, (3) fundamental in developing good standards of care and (4) functional in the development of high-quality research.

In the definition of suicide-related behaviour offered by O'Carroll *et al.* (1996, p. 247), they make the point that there are two aspects to be considered. These are: (1) evidence that the person intended to kill him or herself or (2) evidence that the person wished to use the appearance of killing him or herself in order to attain some other end. A similar view is held here in that suicide-related behaviour does not always mean that the person is suicidal or has tried to kill him or herself. Put simply, there are many behaviours that are related to suicide but which do not end in suicide. For example, either cutting one's wrists or ingesting an overdose of prescribed medication frequently ends in the death of the person. However, some people use the same behaviours to attain a goal other than suicide. Thus, it would seem that similar behaviours could have different meanings. In this book, the term suicide-related behaviour is viewed as a general term that encompasses any behaviour, including verbal cues, that suggests that a person is thinking about suicide or intends to harm or kill him or herself. The sub-division, which involves the person's intention to harm or kill him or herself is summarized in Figure 3.1.

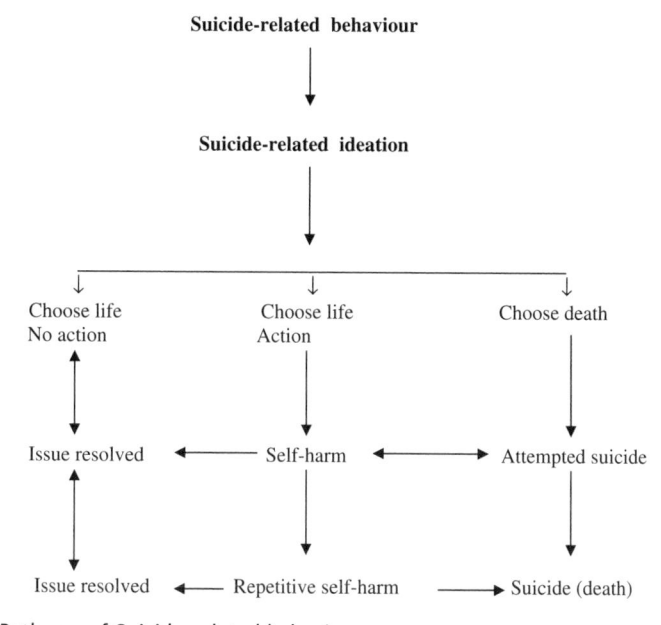

Fig. 3.1 Pathway of Suicide-related behaviour.

Figure 3.1 summarises the pathways of suicide-related behaviour. Each of the terms are briefly defined below and explained in more depth in the following chapter.

- **Suicide-related behaviour:** This is a very general term that includes all self-inflicted life-threatening behaviours including verbal comment in which there is either clear or implied evidence that a person intended or intends to either harm or kill him or herself and which could, whether intentional or not, result in the person's death.
- **Suicide-related ideation:** Where the person reports any thoughts of suicide or self-harm. It will also include any behaviour, whether verbal or non-verbal that could be interpreted as communicating or suggesting that a suicide-related behaviour may occur in the near future.

Death-orientated suicide-related behaviour

- **Attempted suicide:** Any self-harming and potentially life-threatening behaviour with a non-fatal outcome where there is either clear or implied evidence that the harm was self-inflicted and that the person was prepared to die or intended at some non-zero level to kill him or herself.
- **Suicide:** Death from any self-harming and potentially life-threatening behaviour where there is either clear or implied evidence that the behaviour was self-inflicted and that the person was prepared to die or intended at some non-zero level to kill him or herself.

Life-orientated suicide-related behaviour

- **Self-harm:** Any self-harming and potentially life-threatening behaviour with a non-fatal outcome where there is either clear or implied evidence that the harm was self-inflicted but where there was no intention to kill him or herself.
- **Repetitive self-harm:** Any self-harming and potentially life-threatening behaviour with a non-fatal outcome where there is either clear or implied evidence that the harm was self-inflicted but where there was no intention to kill him or herself and which the person has engaged in on more than one occasion.

Inherent in each of these definitions is the person's intention to live or their intention to die at the time of the behaviour. There are well-known difficulties in measuring a person's intention to live or die. A prime reason for this difficulty is that a person's intention is a very personal form of motivation. However, a person can talk about their intention during an interview and the practitioner can interpret the response as being either an explicit or subjective intention. Would a person hint or even talk about wanting to kill or physically harm him or herself if they did not mean it? In trying to answer this question, the practitioner needs to consider the person's past responses to psychological trauma or previous statements that have hinted or suggested that suicide or self-harm was being considered. Thus, in order to clarify a person's intention to live or die, a practitioner needs to consider other available information. In order to help practitioners to elicit a person's intention, Beck and Lester (1976), Beck, Schuyler and Herman (1974), Beck, Kovacs and Weissman (1979) and Pierce (1977) all offer insights into assessing a person's suicidal intent.

Summary

The focus in this chapter was clearly on the type of terminology that is currently used by practitioners when considering the concept of suicide-related behaviour. There are numerous terms that are used to define what suicide is and even more terms are used to define similar behaviours that do not result in suicide. Some of these terms can lead to confusion and misinterpretation among practitioners. Indeed, this is very much a global issue. There is thus the need to limit the number of terms, simplify their meanings and make sense of them in terms of the person's intention. In doing so, this chapter acknowledges the good work by O'Carroll *et al.* (1996) and draws heavily on their nomenclature in order to compress the multitude of terms into a simpler and more tangible form that practitioners can relate to. In addition, the update provided by Silverman (2005, 2006) suggests that the debate is continuing but that obstacles still remain. It is asserted here that the same obstacles have been there and are still there. Nonetheless, the debate on terminology has developed in excess of 50 years, and there is now a very real need to move swiftly towards a common set of terms that represent the range of suicide-related behaviours. Through Figure 3.1, this chapter has attempted to do this and each of the terms used will now be explored in the next chapter.

The concept of suicide-related behaviour

4

In Chapter 4, the following issues are explored:

1. What is suicide-related behaviour?
2. Understanding suicide-related ideation
3. Understanding attempted suicide
4. Understanding suicide
5. Understanding self-harm
6. Repetitive self-harm

What is suicide-related behaviour?

Suicide-related behaviour is very much a global phenomenon and there is evidence of increased rates of suicide found to be emerging across the globe (WHO, 2002a). In addition, the incidences of other similarly related behaviour, such as self-harm, that have the potential to end in suicide, show no sign of declining. An analysis of the definition of suicide-related behaviour indicates that it is a very broad concept. It includes any life-threatening thought or behaviour that suggests that the person intends either to harm or kill him or herself. When a person intends to harm him or herself and does not intend to kill him or herself, then it could be argued that the person has chosen a life option. In contrast, when a person intends to die, then it is very easy to argue that they have chosen a death option. So why should we use the term suicide-related behaviour? Well, let us consider a fictionally based case history with different outcomes in the next four case vignettes and discuss some of the issues.

Case vignette 16

Herbert was 19 years of age and had been in a relationship with Jenny for two years. Both of them were now in their second year in university doing separate courses. In the last few months he had grown very fond of her and he had begun to plan their future together. Initially Jenny was very much for the idea but in the last few months she wanted to do other things and did not want the same commitment. This upset Herbert and he had become very depressed in the last few weeks. His vision of their being together in the future had been shattered. He tried talking to Jenny on a number of occasions but the more he tried to convince her to stay the more she wanted to be just friends. He let her and some close friends know that he no longer cared whether he lived or died. One night Herbert and Jenny had another row and she told him that she wanted to go out with other males. Herbert stormed off. In the morning his parents found him in the bathroom in a collapsed state. He had cut both his wrists. He was rushed to hospital but unfortunately Herbert was pronounced dead on arrival at hospital.

Discussion point: In a small group of fellow students, spend 10–15 minutes discussing your interpretation of Herbert's death in Case vignette 16. Think of the terms in Boxes 3.1–3.3 that you are familiar with and decide what you would call Herbert's behaviour. Would you categorize this case vignette as suicide-related behaviour? Write down your rationale for your decisions and compare them with other students.

Case vignette 17

Herbert was 19 years of age and had been in a relationship with Jenny for two years. Both of them were now in their second year in university doing separate courses. In the last few months he had grown very fond of her and he had begun to plan their future together. Initially Jenny was very much for the idea but in the last few months she wanted to do other things and did not want the same commitment. This upset Herbert and he had become very depressed in the last few weeks. His vision of their being together in the future had been shattered. He tried talking to Jenny on a number of occasions but the more he tried to convince her to stay the more she wanted to be just friends. He let her and some close friends know that he no longer cared whether he lived or died. One night Herbert and Jenny had another row and she said that she wanted to go out with other males. Herbert stormed off. In the morning his parents found him in the bathroom in a collapsed state. He had cut both his wrists. He was rushed to the Accident and Emergency Department of the local hospital where he had an infusion of blood, his wounds were dressed and he eventually made a full recovery.

Discussion point: In a small group of fellow students spend 10–15 minutes discussing your interpretation of Herbert's behaviour in Case vignette 17. Think of the terms in Boxes 3.1–3.3 that you are familiar with and decide what you would call Herbert's behaviour. Would you categorize this case vignette as suicide-related behaviour? Write down your rationale for your decisions and compare them with other students.

Case vignette 18

Herbert was 19 years of age and had been in a relationship with Jenny for two years. Both of them were now in their second year in university doing separate courses. In the last few months he had grown very fond of her and he had begun to plan their future together. Initially Jenny was very much for the idea but in the last few months she wanted to do other things and did not want the same commitment. This upset Herbert and he had become very depressed in the last few weeks. His vision of their being together in the future had been shattered. He tried talking to Jenny on a number of occasions but the more he tried to convince her to stay the more she wanted to be just friends. One night Herbert and Jenny had another row and she said that she wanted to go out with other males. Herbert stormed off. In the morning his parents found him in the bathroom in a collapsed state. He had cut both his wrists. He was rushed to the Accident and Emergency Department of the local hospital where he had an infusion of blood, his wounds were dressed and he eventually made a full recovery.

Discussion point: In a small group of fellow students spend 10–15 minutes discussing your interpretation of Herbert's behaviour in Case vignette 18. Think of the terms in Boxes 3.1–3.3 that you are familiar with and decide what you would call Herbert's behaviour. Would you categorize this case vignette as suicide-related behaviour? Write down your rationale for your decisions and compare them with other students.

Case vignette 19

Herbert is 20 years of age. Currently he is living on his own in an apartment. He previously attended accident and emergency nine months ago after cutting both his wrists. On that occasion he and his girlfriend had broken up. Yesterday, after failing a number of assignments, he was informed by his university teachers that his work was not up to scratch and that he was in danger of having to withdraw from the course. Following this news he went to his apartment and cut his wrists. However, he cut too deeply and he was concerned that he had done serious damage. He immediately dressed his wounds and went to the Accident and Emergency Department of the local hospital.

Discussion point: In a small group of fellow students spend 10–15 minutes discussing your interpretation of Herbert's behaviour in Case vignette 19. Think of the terms in Boxes 3.1–3.3 that you are familiar with and decide what you would call Herbert's behaviour. Would you categorize this case vignette as suicide-related behaviour? Write down your rationale for your decisions and compare them with other students.

You will of course have noted that the reason why Herbert cut his wrists is the same in vignettes 16–18. However, there is a different reason in Case vignette 19. Nonetheless, if you analyse what happened in Case vignette 16 you will find that Herbert was ambivalent about life and death. He had let Jenny and some close friends know that he did not care whether he lived or died. As a result, Herbert performed a life-threatening behaviour that resulted in his death. In this case vignette, one could argue that it was suicide. The term suicide is reserved for those who kill themselves and where there is evidence that the person intended at some level to die. Some people may say that Herbert's expression of suicidal intent was very low. However, the fact remains that he did say it and thus people were given due notice of his suicidal intent. Therefore, Herbert's death, while still coming as a shock to those in whom he confided, could have been foreseen and possibly prevented. In contrast, in Case vignette 17 Herbert was still ambivalent about life and death but he managed to survive after cutting his wrists. How would you term this? It certainly would not be called suicide. Again, one must go back to Herbert's previously expressed ambivalence about life and death. While one could argue that this represents an expression of low suicide intent, it is still an expression of suicide intent and therefore above the non-zero level. As such, the term 'attempted suicide' would seem to be the most appropriate.

However, in Case vignette 18 Herbert did not indicate any intention of harming or killing himself but for the same reasons he cuts his wrists and he again survives. If you and your group came to the conclusion that Herbert's wrist-cutting in Case vignette 18 could be termed self-harm, then you could be right – or you could be very wrong. Even though Herbert did not express any intention of harm or death, an in-depth assessment of his suicide intention at the time he cut his wrists and an assessment of his risk of future suicide would need to be carried out. By doing this, you would then be able to find out information that may have a direct effect on Herbert's future care needs. In what seems to be a contrast, Case vignette 19 gives a different reason why Herbert cut his wrists. Also, and similar to Case vignette 18, he had given no warning to family or friends about his intentions. However, there is a possibility that Herbert had learned from his previous experience and now his cutting behaviour may be the beginning of using self-harm as a coping measure. Unfortunately, there is little evidence to support this assertion and an in-depth assessment will be necessary to ascertain Herbert's intention at the time he cut his wrists.

If you are of the opinion that the behaviours in each of the four case vignettes above are related to suicide and that the main differences between them are: (1) Herbert's intention to live or die; and (2) outcomes (life and death), then you would be right. Herbert's behaviour could have resulted in his death in all four case vignettes. We have got to remember that according to its definition, suicide-related behaviour can include a wide range of behaviours such as verbal cues or other more physical behaviours which indicate that a person is thinking, at some non-zero level, about suicide or that they intended to harm or kill him or herself. In each of Herbert's four case vignettes, this has been so.

In this chapter, consideration is given to those specific terms that were defined earlier as falling within the general term of suicide-related behaviour. These specific terms are: (1) suicide-related ideation; (2) attempted suicide; (3) suicide; (4) self-harm; (5) repetitive self-harm.

Understanding suicide-related ideation

Some practitioners will argue that suicide-related ideation should not be included as part of suicide-related behaviour. It is asserted here that thinking about suicide or self-harm is very much a part of suicide-related behaviour and as such should be included in the concept. In much the same way that cognitive therapy and behavioural therapy can be linked together, similarly thinking about self-harm or suicide can be linked to suicide-related behaviour. What type of events lead to suicide-related ideation? The answer to this question will be more specifically dealt with in the next few chapters. However, a few brief examples are mentioned here. This brief list is neither exclusive nor exhaustive but serves to illustrate some main reasons why people may consider suicide-related behaviour. For example, loneliness (Stravynski and Boyer, 2001), feelings of hopelessness (Pinto, Whisman and Conwell, 1998; Abramson et al., 1998; Barbe et al., 2004), psychiatric illnesses such as depression (Brádvik, 2003), isolation or social exclusion (Bowler, 2001), and difficulties in interpersonal relationships (Hawton et al., 2000; DoH, 2001).

Sometimes when a person indicates that they are considering a suicide-related behaviour at some time in the future, it may seem like a suicide threat. This is true. In fact, suicide threat (see Box 3.1) is a term that is used by some practitioners. The application of such a term towards a person who has indicated that they are considering some form of suicide-related behaviour can create negative attitudes in others. For this reason the term 'suicide threat' is not an acceptable term and it seems that other authors such as Dear (1997) share this viewpoint. In this book, it is affirmed that the term suicide-related ideation adequately covers all of the similar terms that have been presented in Box 3.1, including 'suicide threat'. Put simply, the person has expressed either verbally or by other means that they are considering some form of suicide-related behaviour. Rarely does suicide-related ideation arise out of the blue and more than likely it is in response to some stressor in a person's life. The only care responses that practitioners can employ are to explore why the person feels the way they do and secondly to find out the person's risk of future suicide. Indeed, Morgan and Stanton (1997) concluded by emphasizing the importance of monitoring suicide-related ideation when assessing the risk of future suicide. The definition of suicide-related ideation that is used here builds on the definition that was used by O'Carroll *et al.* (1996): 'Suicide-related ideation is where the person reports any thoughts of suicide or self-harm. It will also include any behaviour, whether verbal or non-verbal that could be interpreted as communicating or suggesting that a suicide-related behaviour may occur in the near future.'

When a person is considering some form of suicide-related behaviour as an option, they have usually, but not always, reached a crisis point. Not only does it include the person's verbally expressed thoughts but it will also include any observed behaviour that could suggest that the person is thinking about suicide-related behaviour. Indeed suicide-related ideation would include any thoughts that range from vague ideas about the possibility of suicide to actually making plans to die by suicide at some time in the future. In addition, some people, for the same reasons, may think about self-harm as a strategy for alleviating distress and emotional despair. For example, think about Herbert's Case vignette 19 above. He may not have verbally expressed any suicide-related behaviour but there is some evidence that he has thought about it. In an effort to get help, many people will give early warning signs to family, friends, clergy or other similar professionals (Rankin, 1989; LivingWorks, 2004). These early warning signs may on occasion be very obvious. However, more often than not they are very subtle negative comments that are very general and suggest little hope for the future. For example, when a person is thinking about suicide they may say things like:

1. 'It will soon be over anyway!'
2. 'What's the point of living? '
3. 'I wish I was dead.'
4. 'Nobody will miss me when I am gone!'
5. 'I will not be needing these things any more.'

In addition, the behaviour of some people may change from their normal pattern prior to their suicide. For instance, some people may make their last will and testament and sort out financial and other such affairs. Other people may give away personal and possibly valuable belongings. They may visit family and friends whom they have not seen for a while. Also, it has long been known that many of those who kill themselves visit their GPs prior to their suicide (Bancroft et al.,1977; Kreitman, 1989; Vassilas and Morgan, 1993; Stenager and Jensen, 1994; DHSSPSNI, 2006). Unfortunately, when talking to their GP, many will mask their suicide-related ideation with vague physiological symptoms (Chin, Touquet and Burns, 1986). Also, Stenager and Jensen (1994) found that almost 54% of people, who had suicide-related ideation, at the time of their last GP consultation, did not tell their GP about them. From these reports, it would seem that suicide-related ideation is more associated with adults. However, Sorenson and Rutter (1991) found that 11.7% of children reported suicide-related ideation but not any overt suicide-related behaviour. Thus, it seems that suicide-related ideation can occur in all age groups. While one person talks to the Samaritans about suicide every minute in the day in the UK and Ireland (Samaritans, 2006), it is not known how many people talk to other professionals involved in health care or to support workers and lay people about their suicidal thoughts. For example, let us consider Case vignette 20.

Case vignette 20

I recall an incident on a cold winter's night when I was in the company of a very good friend of mine who was also a member of the clergy. We were in deep discussion about religion and spirituality. At about 11.30 p.m. his doorbell rang and the housekeeper answered. He was called away but asked me to wait. About one hour later he appeared. He told me that a middle-aged lady had been on her way to kill herself by drowning and that she planned to jump off the local pier. As she passed by his house she noticed that there was a light on in his office. On the spur of the moment she called in to talk to him. At the end of their talk he persuaded her to make a promise to him that she would go home and call to see him the following afternoon. Afterwards, in talking to me he did two things:

1. He maintained the anonymity of the person.
2. He began to talk in general about the number of people who had called to see him about their suicidal thoughts.

He expressed his concern that there were a growing number of people who called to him for help and that he had no training whatsoever in dealing with people who wanted to kill or harm themselves. He asked me about his actions and I reassured him that his action with the lady would demonstrate to her that someone cared. For instance, it would give her a reason to live until the following afternoon and it would allow her time to consider, review and possibly revise her plans to kill herself.

Case vignette 21

In another incident, a lady called June (pseudonym) asked to see me as she was concerned about her husband's mental well-being. She told me that her husband's friend had killed himself a few months earlier. It seemed that prior to the suicide the friend had indicated to June's husband his intention to kill himself. However, the husband disbelieved it and brushed the thought off. When the friend killed himself, the husband thought that he could have prevented it but had failed to do so. In effect, he blamed himself for his friend's death. In relating her story, June was aware that her husband felt guilty about his friend's death. She felt that her husband was blaming himself too much and she also thought that he was considering suicide as a result of this guilt. June was worried about this and did not know how to broach this with her husband. We worked out a plan and we role-played a potential situation between her and her husband. June played herself and I played her husband. At an appropriate time she raised her concern with her husband. June came to see me the week after this and told me that her husband was stunned by her analysis and he admitted that he was considering suicide and did not know how to talk to her or anyone else about it. He immediately felt relieved that June had brought up the topic and that he could now talk openly with her about his feelings and his rationale for wanting to die. June informed me that following their discussions her husband was thinking about joining a local group who gave support to those bereaved by suicide.

Case vignette 22

In another example Mark came to see me as he was thinking about killing himself. However, he had not acted on these thoughts. Prior to these thoughts, Mark had established his own business and even though he was only in his mid twenties, he had become quite successful. One day after an important and very successful business lunch with a client, Mark had been stopped driving by the police and a breath test found that his alcohol intake was over the legal limit. He was charged with drunken driving and was expecting a court appearance in the near future. He lived with his elderly parents and his younger siblings. He thought that his elderly parents would be unable to cope with his impending conviction and the resultant family shame. In addition, he felt that he had been a terrible example to his younger siblings. By the time he sought help Mark was in a high state of anxiety. He could not consider talking to his parents because of his own feelings of shame and he had thought about suicide. He could not see any other options that might resolve the difficulties he was facing. Mark went to his GP to talk to him about his feelings and also to find out if his GP would arrange to test a sample of his blood. Regarding the blood testing, his GP told him to seek an independent laboratory to have it tested. Unfortunately, he did not know of any. Nonetheless, his GP did listen to his story but informed Mark that there was nothing he could do about his impending court case. His verbal response to Mark was, 'I know it is cold comfort, but it might help you to settle if you took some of these (Anxiolytic) tablets'. Mark reluctantly agreed and he was given a prescription for a drug from the benzodiazepine group. However, while Mark knew his GP felt and showed concern, he also recognized that his GP did not have the time to help him. Also, he felt that the medication would only allay his physical symptoms and would do little to alleviate his emotional worries.

Mark sought additional help to work through his feelings and it was at this point that we met. He told me all about the events leading up to our point of contact. This included his thoughts about using the tablets his GP prescribed to kill himself. Through discussion, we explored his feelings about the drink-driving charge, his impending court appearance and his suicidal thoughts. Eventually, Mark came to the conclusion that his major stressor was not the impending court case but the thought of telling his elderly parents about what happened. He decided that he would have to tell them sooner rather than later. Having reached that decision we discussed the pros and cons of different scenarios in which he could talk to his parents. Eventually we chose and role-played several scenarios. When he felt confident about it, he then talked to his parents, went to court and paid his debt to society. About a year later Mark asked to see me again. At this meeting he told me that he had regained his driving licence after six months and that his business was currently making good progress. He also informed me that he no longer drank alcohol during business lunches.

From these case histories it seems that a number of people consider the possibility of suicide as an option when faced with difficulties in their lives and there is evidence that suicide-related ideation is positively linked with negative life events, help-seeking behaviours, self-harm and attempted suicide (Goldney et al., 1989; Reinherz et al., 1995; Wilson et al., 1995; Adams and Adams, 1996; Metha and McWhirter, 1997; O'Sullivan and Ftizgerald, 1998; Kessler, Borges and Walters, 1999; Lawlor and James, 2000; Carlton and Deane, 2000; Rowly, Ganter and Fitzpatrick, 2001; Stravynski and Boyer, 2001; Dunham, 2004). It has even been reported that many top names in the entertainment industry have thought about suicide and in some cases have attempted suicide (Levine, 2005).

Each of these previous case histories, as well as quite a few other similar case studies and the reports from organizations such as the Samaritans, strongly suggest that many people consider suicide-related behaviour as an option. In addition, many professional people, other than those who are directly involved in the mental health caring services, come into contact with people who express suicide-related ideation: for example, the clergy, teachers, community volunteers, and people who are considered as support workers. Therefore, it can be assumed that the actual number of people who think about suicide is much larger than the number reported as doing so. Unfortunately, there is no accurate method by which it would be possible to record all those who express suicide-related ideation.

What are the outcomes of suicide-related ideation? Well, there are a number of potential outcomes. For instance, the person can choose to: (1) take no further action or (2) seek help as in the case of Mark or June's case histories as outlined above. In both case vignettes the help-seeking behaviour averted potential suicide-related behaviour. However, a person in distress or who is experiencing despair may choose to act very differently and that action could result in serious harm or quite possibly their death. An alternative outcome focuses on suicide and revolves around some statistics with which we are familiar. For instance, as mentioned earlier, we know that in the United Kingdom (UK) the Samaritans receive a call from someone who is thinking about suicide approximately every minute of every day. Also, in the UK, one person kills themselves approximately every two hours. Over a period of a year, the number of suicides in the UK will account for only 1% of the number of people who express thoughts about suicide. From these approximations, one could argue that most of the people who think about suicide can transform their thoughts of suicide and do not go on to kill themselves. This information is very useful and offers some degree of hope for most people who express thoughts about suicide. In addition, Shea (2002) suggested that for most people thoughts about suicide are transient in nature. However, Shea (2002) also adds that there is a good chance of helping those whose thoughts about suicide are known, but this means that practitioners need to uncover the suicidal ideations first.

Understanding attempted suicide

The most significant part of the definition of attempted suicide is that the person was prepared to die or intended, at some level, to die. This suggests that there may be different levels of intention. For instance, it could be concluded that for those who attempt suicide, some will have had a very high intention of killing themselves and some will have had a very low intention of killing themselves. In fact some authors suggest that the intention to kill oneself is low in some cases of suicide-related behaviour (Arensman and Kerkhof, 1996; Hawton *et al.*, 2004). The difficulty with using terms such as low suicide intent, is that some practitioners may interpret a potentially life-threatening behaviour where there is 'low suicide intent' as self-harm rather than attempted suicide. The nettle that practitioners need to grasp here is that whenever there is any intention, whether regarded as high or low, of killing oneself, then it must be interpreted as attempted suicide. Irrespective of whether the person's intention was high or low, there is every possibility that their suicide-related behaviour failed by chance rather than by choice. To label the suicide-related behaviour anything else may miss the point and may have an impact on how practitioners should interact with the person.

As mentioned earlier, Shneidman (1985) and Dear (1997) both explore ambivalence as being common in suicide-related behaviour. In addition, Dear (1997) also makes the point that both: (1) being ambivalent about life and death and (2) being prepared to die are above the non-zero level. In agreement with Dear (1997) it is asserted here that all suicide-related behaviour where there is evidence of low suicide intent should be classified as attempted suicide and not as any form of self-harm. This may be anathema to some practitioners and there is current debate on the topic. However, many health care practitioners will note that the point being made here is to tease out the differences between 'attempted suicide' on one hand and 'self-harm' on the other. To suggest that both are the same is to perpetuate the confusion that has existed for far too many years.

It is fairly well accepted that the term suicide involves death from any behaviour such as injury, poisoning or suffocation and where there is implicit or explicit evidence that the behaviour was self-inflicted and that the person intended to kill himself/herself. When those conditions all apply, there is no doubt that the outcome must be termed suicide. However, what happens when all those conditions apply but the outcome does not result in death? For example, when there is either implicit or explicit evidence that the behaviour was self- inflicted and that the person intended to kill himself/herself but the person survived. Practitioners can only determine that, irrespective of the type of behaviour used or the lethality of that behaviour, the person tried to kill him or herself. Behaviour that meets all the criteria for suicide but which does not result in death can only be referred to as 'attempted suicide'.

As mentioned earlier the excess of terms currently used means that it is difficult to estimate the numbers of people who attempt suicide (O'Carroll *et al.,* 1996; Hjelmeland *et al.,* 2000). A recent consultation document on the Northern Ireland suicide prevention strategy (DHSSPSNI, 2006) focuses mainly on suicide and also discusses self-harm. However, it does not overtly address 'attempted suicide' and there are no statistics to suggest how many persons were admitted to hospital following an attempted suicide. It is very possible that many of those reported as having self-harmed should have been more accurately described as 'attempted suicide'. The inclusion of low suicide intent in the definition of attempted suicide would substantially reduce the numbers of those admitted to hospital following self-harm. What is more, such an inclusion would also increase the numbers of persons recorded as having 'attempted suicide'. There is a very strong possibility that Professor Hawton and colleagues in the Centre for Suicide Research in Oxford (UK) had got it right. For many years they opted to use the term attempted suicide to describe most such admissions. It is quite possible that there were many people who when they first performed some form of suicide-related behaviour did actually attempt to kill themselves. For instance, McLaughlin, Miller and Warwick (1996) reported that 14 of their respondents stated that their self-harm would influence their problem because they would be dead. They also add that this group of respondents scored significantly higher on hopelessness and depression. Based on what the authors report, it seems that this group of respondents attempted suicide rather than self-harmed. Another example is that, in Stephen's case history (Case vignette 4), at the time of his suicide-related behaviour his intention was to die and on assessment he did score quite high on the Suicide Intent Scale as described by Beck, Schuyler and Herman (1974). However, Stephen's survival did have a restraining and preventative effect on any future suicide-related behaviour. It is quite possible that this happens in many other similar cases. For instance, Levine (2005) describes the suicide attempts of a number of stars from the world of entertainment. In some cases it seems that their suicide attempt did have a restraining effect on future suicide attempts. However, for some people unresolved issues could result in either another attempt with a fatal outcome (suicide) or the development of self-harm as a coping measure.

I have no doubt that a number of practitioners will criticize the term 'attempted suicide'. For example, Silverman (2005) makes a very valid point that the term 'attempted suicide' suggests failure on the part of the person. There is a possibility that the use of the term 'attempted suicide' may impact on the person's evaluation of his or her own behaviour. For instance, from a cognitive therapy point of view it is possible that the term 'attempted suicide' may reinforce, in the person, already negative thinking by adding in a new self-evaluation such as 'I am so useless that I can't even kill myself.' Nevertheless, when there is no doubt that the person did try to kill him or herself, then the truth must be told: that is what happened – the person attempted to kill themselves. No matter whether a person's intention to kill him or herself was high or low, it is very possible that they will try to kill themselves again (Isometsa and Lonnqvist, 1998). This possibility has implications for therapeutic care required by people who have tried to kill themselves. For instance, a very important step in the therapeutic relationship is that the practitioner must affirm and acknowledge the person's psychache or emotional despair. Not acknowledging the seriousness of the person's attempt to kill themselves could create a barrier between the practitioner and the person. For instance, if the practitioner strongly suspects that the person is thinking about suicide then they should acknowledge it as such (LivingWorks, 2004). A similar acknowledgement should be applied where there is evidence that the person has attempted to kill him or herself.

At this stage it is quite obvious that the assessment of a person's psychological needs is of the utmost importance. Part of such an assessment would, in the case of suicide-related behaviour, include an assessment of future suicide risk. This is one of the primary reasons why the term 'attempted suicide' is used in this book. As stated earlier, for those who have attempted suicide, there is a very real risk that they will try to kill themselves at some stage in the future. Unfortunately, a major hazard, which can complicate an accurate suicide risk assessment in the clinical environment, would include misleading clinical improvement, and reluctance on the part of the person to discuss their suicidal thoughts (Morgan and Stanton, 1997). It is very difficult to accept but the Department of Health (2001) reported that in their analysis between 25% and 30% of persons killed themselves within three months of discharge from hospital. Therefore, it is emphasized here that a previous history of attempted suicide in a person indicates a high risk of future suicide. Also, and very importantly, when the practitioner has evidence to support their thoughts, they need to acknowledge not only the severity of a person's emotional pain and distress, but also the fact that they tried to kill themselves.

Understanding suicide

Quite a number of practitioners would agree that suicide is a long-term solution to a short-term difficulty. This may seem like an old cliché; however all practitioners must acknowledge that suicide is a solution and is a popular option chosen by approximately 5000 people in the United Kingdom and Ireland each year. It may not be the correct solution, but it is a very permanent solution. Recently the Samaritans (2006) released their analysis of suicide trends over the last 10 years. Their analysis shows that in the United Kingdom there has been a 9.5% decrease overall. However, much of this is accounted for by the 11% decrease in suicides in England and the 15% decrease in suicides in Wales. While there has been a 1% increase in suicides in Scotland, the trends in Northern Ireland remained fairly static. In contrast, there was a 13% increase in suicides in the Republic of Ireland over the 10 year period. Methods that are used to kill oneself vary and can involve any type of behaviour. However, the main methods that are recorded are given in Box 4.1.

In Box 4.1, the methods of suicide that are identified are not exclusive as people can choose any method. While the method chosen in most female suicides is overdosing, most male suicides are by hanging. Unfortunately and for whatever reason it seems that alternative solutions to the person's life difficulties seem to be unavailable or are not foreseeable at the time of the person's suicide. However, more often than not, the difficulties faced by the person could have had an alternative solution. For this reason, it is very possible that of all the causes of death, suicide is probably the most tragic and the most difficult to understand. According

Box 4.1   Methods used in suicide.

Hanging
Overdosing
Shooting
Drowning
Cutting
Jumping from high structures
Crashing a vehicle

Table 4.1   Comparison of rates per 100 000 population aged 15 years+ for suicide and undetermined deaths for both males and females.

Year	England	Northern Ireland	Wales	Ireland (ROI)	Scotland
1998	13.59	13.37	14.82	19.70	20.80
1999	13.29	13.40	15.62	17.93	20.70
2000	12.96	15.22	14.48	18.60	20.77
2001	12.80	11.97	13.33	19.67	20.93
2002	10.97	15.25	12.87	16.21	21.20
Mean rate	12.72	13.84	14.22	18.42	20.88

Data in Table 4.1 was supplied by the Northern Ireland Statistics and Research Agency, Central Statistics Office (Ireland), Office of National Statistics (England and Wales); General Registrar Office (Scotland).

to the World Health Organization approximately 849 000 people died as a result of suicide during 2001 (WHO, 2002b). Furthermore, there is a very real possibility that the number of persons killing themselves will increase each year. In Table 4.1, during the years 1998–2002 an analysis of the raw number of recorded suicides in the United Kingdom (UK) and in Ireland shows that when male and female suicides are combined, there is a decrease in the rate of recorded suicide in England and in Wales but that recorded suicides in Northern Ireland and in Scotland indicate an increasing trend. However, when the mean is examined over the five-year period, one can see that England has the lowest rate and that Scotland has the highest rate.

When these statistics are teased out into the rates of male suicides for each country, Table 4.2 shows that for males, England, Wales and Ireland have a

Table 4.2 Comparison of rates per 100 000 population aged 15 years+ for suicide and undetermined deaths for males.

Year	England	Northern Ireland	Wales	Ireland (ROI)	Scotland
1998	21.37	20.58	22.86	33.12	32.44
1999	20.83	21.66	26.05	28.42	32.82
2000	19.98	24.69	23.92	30.17	33.36
2001	19.47	20.33	22.63	32.52	32.22
2002	16.84	24.48	21.55	26.60	33.60
Mean rate	19.70	22.34	23.40	30.17	32.89

Data in Table 4.2 was supplied by the Northern Ireland Statistics and Research Agency, Central Statistics Office (Ireland), Office of National Statistics (England and Wales); General Registrar Office (Scotland).

Table 4.3 Comparison of rates per 100 000 population aged 15 years+ for suicide and undetermined deaths for females.

Year	Wales	Northern Ireland	England	Ireland (ROI)	Scotland
1998	7.47	6.7	6.40	6.72	10.22
1999	6.06	5.77	6.33	7.77	8.79
2000	5.86	6.47	6.02	7.38	9.15
2001	4.87	4.23	6.61	7.18	10.78
2002	4.98	6.67	5.46	6.12	10.00
Mean rate	5.85	5.97	6.16	7.03	9.788

Data in Table 4.3 was supplied by the Northern Ireland Statistics and Research Agency, Central Statistics Office (Ireland), Office of National Statistics (England and Wales); General Registrar Office (Scotland).

decreasing trend. However, the rates of suicide per 100 000 population for Northern Ireland and for Scotland indicate an increasing trend.

When these statistics are teased out into the rates of female suicides for each country, Table 4.3 shows that for females, England, Wales and Ireland have a decreasing trend. However, the rates of suicide per 100 000 population for Northern Ireland and for Scotland indicate an increasing trend.

What is particularly striking about these statistics is that they show that the annual rate of suicide for males is almost four times greater than it is for females.

Also, while the rate of female suicide remains fairly static for each country, it is very noticeable that the rate of female suicide is considerably higher for Scotland than for any other country in the United Kingdom or in the Republic of Ireland. This point is also borne out in a recent report from Northern Ireland, which analysed the rate of suicide during the period 1991–2003. For instance, this document shows that the rate of male suicide in Northern Ireland is increasing but that the rate of female suicide has remained fairly constant during the period (Information Analysis Directorate, 2006). This information may be reassuring to females. However, Zahl and Hawton (2004) make the point that while most male suicides are successful on first attempt, females are more likely to be successful on second attempts. Therefore, just because the annual suicide rate is lower for females than it is for males, there is no room for complacency.

Attempted suicide and suicide are both death-orientated behaviours. As stated earlier, there is a very real chance that, if not responded to in an appropriate way, a person who has survived a suicide attempt may eventually go on to kill themselves. Why might people go on to kill themselves? This question will be explored in more detail in Chapter 5 ('The descent into crisis'). However, it must be said here that there is no one reason why people would want to kill themselves. Furthermore, the main reasons why people want to kill themselves involve loss of some kind. The person's interpretation of the loss and how it impacts on them is central to their reasons for killing themselves. These same reasons are applicable to those people who have attempted suicide. Therefore, the main suggestion here is that attempted suicide and suicide are very much interlinked and intertwined.

Understanding self-harm

From the outset, it is important to point out that in the academic literature self-harm is frequently confused with attempted suicide, but there should be no confusion. Self-harm is not the same as attempted suicide (Muehlenkamp and Gutierrez, 2004) nor is it a subset of suicide. However, and very much at odds with what has just been stated, it is true that those who self-harm are very much at high risk of eventual suicide. Therefore, there is a definite relationship between self-harm and suicide. For instance there is a growing body of knowledge to suggest that people self-harm in order to avoid killing themselves (Connors, 1996; Babiker and Arnold, 1997; Pembroke, 1998a, 1998b, 1998c). Why do people choose to harm themselves? The simple answer is that there are many reasons why people would want to harm themselves. However, the most general over-reaching reason why a person would self-harm is that (s)he has reached breaking point while trying to cope with their emotional despair. The occurrence of self-harm is very suggestive that the person's previous coping strategies, such as verbal expression of their suicide-related ideation or other less obvious behaviour, have proved to be ineffective. As a possible result of ineffective support or in the absence of any support, self-harm can become the person's coping response to their difficulties. According to the definition of self-harm made earlier, there will be clear or implied evidence that the person inflicted the harm but that (s)he had no intention of dying. Self-harm behaviour can include a wide range of behaviours and includes all forms of self-poisoning and self-injury (Zahl and Hawton, 2004). However, some practitioners may take issue with this as their experience of working with people in distress leads them to believe that there is a distinct difference between those who injure themselves and those who poison themselves. I would state categorically that I agree totally that there is a difference in both behaviours. However, I have to add that my reason for including both under the same umbrella of self-harm is that in both cases it is not the behaviour that is of importance, it is the underlying reasons why they self-harm.

Discussion points:

1. In a small group of fellow students spend about 10 minutes drawing up a list of the methods people would use to self-harm. Compare your list with other students.

2. In a small group of fellow students spend about 10 minutes drawing up a list of reasons why a person would self-harm. Compare your list and reasons with other students.

The definition of self-harm does not imply an intention to die. The self-harm act frequently follows a psychological crisis (Klerman, 1987) and most such crises are short-lived (Waterhouse and Platt, 1990). Also, Hawton and Catalan (1987) suggest that two-thirds of those who self-harm may think about the act for less than an hour beforehand. In Europe, cited self-harm rates for males range from 45 to 314 per 100 000 population while the rates for females range from 69 to 462 per 100 000 population (Schmidtke *et al.*, 1996). Rates of between 2200 and 3760 per 100 000 inmates have been reported in prisons (Toch, 1975). In a recent report in Northern Ireland (DHSSPSNI, 2006), it was reported that the highest average number of admissions for self-harm per 100 000 persons were in Derry (452.5), and in Belfast (445.5). This report also suggests that the similarity of these findings suggest that self-harm is widespread in Northern Ireland. In addition, they report that the incidence of self-harm is lower in those aged 75 years and over (DHSSPSNI, 2006). Thus, self-harm occurs in most age groups. Also, in Northern Ireland there are approximately 4500 admissions to hospital for self-harm each year (Information Analysis Directorate, 2006). However, in the Republic of Ireland there are approximately 11 000 such admissions each year

(Health Service Executive, 2005). Recently the Mental Health Foundation and the Camelot Foundation published their long-awaited report in which they estimate that self-harm effects 1 in every 15 young people. Overall, there is no shortage of evidence that the incidence of self-harm is very high. In Box 4.2 there are examples of reasons why people self-harm. However, it is important to remember that a person may self-harm for reasons other than those identified in Box 4.2. Therefore, the reasons given in Box 4.2 should be taken as examples only.

The reasons why a person would self-harm are very personal to the person themselves. It has become their personalized coping mechanism. Similarly, the method that a person chooses to self-harm is very personal to them. Indeed, they may have chosen the method for a particular reason or for no particular reason. In a way this is a pointer towards future therapy as it is not the self-harm behaviour that is of most importance but why the person is self-harming that needs to be addressed. However, Box 4.3 gives some examples of the methods that people choose to self-harm.

It has been reported that an increase in suicide in young men has been accompanied by an increase in self-harm among males (Beck *et al.*, 1994; Stark, Smith and Hall, 1994). Also, many of those who self-harm often belong to the social groups associated with social destabilization and poverty (Schmidtke *et al.*, 1996). For example, an earlier report indicated that self-harm in social class V was more than eight times that in social classes I and II (Platt *et al.*, 1988).

In self-harm, it seems that the intentions of some people are not to die but to seek a rest or try to get a respite from their psychache. While reasons why a person would want to self-harm have been given previously, there are other very specific reasons that a person may self-harm and these can be viewed in Box 4.4.

Box 4.2 Examples of why a person would self-harm.

Physical, sexual, or emotional abuse
Loss/separation/parental divorce
Bullying
Personal shame (e.g. sexuality)
Lack of support from others
Poor interpersonal communication skills
Poor problem-solving skills
Abusive relationships (adults)
Parental alcoholism / drug abuse
Rejection by peers
Racism
Imprisonment

Box 4.3   Examples of methods used in self-harm.

Cutting
Fist banging
Overdosing
Scratching
Burning (cigarettes or caustic substance)
Drinking noxious substances
Excessive scrubbing of the skin
Injecting foreign substances into muscles
Head banging (against walls)
Hair pulling (trichotillomania)
Alcohol or drug abuse
Anorexia
Bulimia

Box 4.4   Examples of very specific reasons for self-harm.

- The person may blame him/herself for an event and they want to punish themselves for it.
- To release anger. This could be anger at another person or anger at themselves for some particular reason.
- To communicate their emotional, physical or psychological pain to others.
- To turn their emotional pain into physical pain. It is much easier to deal with physical pain than it is to deal with emotional pain.

One way of getting a respite from their emotional problems is to get some sleep. For example, in order to get this sleep some people may take an overdose of unprescribed tablets or they may take more than the dosage prescribed by their doctor. Keir (1986) makes this point very well when he suggests that many people who take an overdose, without any intention of killing themselves, are quite possibly trying to get some respite from their emotional despair or as Shneidman (1993) suggests their psychache. Drug overdose is by far the most common form of self-harm and taking an overdose seems to be very popular in the adolescent age group with a higher incidence in females (Hawton *et al.*, 2000). Frequently these adolescents have experienced relationship difficulties with friends or family (DoH, 2001), or had difficulties at school or at work (Hawton *et al.*, 1982). Indeed, some 14 years later, Hawton, Fagg and Simkin (1996) and Kerfoot *et al.* (1996) reported similar findings. Also, Evans (1994) suggested a sequential pattern of interpersonal difficulty from early childhood. In addition, it seems that paracetamol is used in most overdoses (Hawton and Fagg, 1992; Hawton, Fagg and Simkin, 1996). However, there is a high possibility that using paracetamol as a method of self-harm may be reduced following the introduction of legislation and restrictions on the availability of paracetamol (Hawton, 2002).

While the intention of some people is to get some sleep, get a break, or escape from their difficulty, the intentions of other people who self-harm may be entirely different. It is very possible that some people may be angry at the way other people treat them and they may be unable to cope with some very traumatic issues in their lives. Alternatively, some people internalize their thoughts and may blame themselves for difficulties in their lives. This type of thinking can result in their devaluing themselves as being less than what they are. For instance an early trend in psychoanalytic thinking was to link Sigmund Freud's (1917/1957) theory of melancholia with the dynamics of depression (Meissner, 1977). Suicide-related behaviour could be linked to Freud's theory concerning the internal conflicts between the demands of the Id on one hand and the demands of the Super-Ego on the other. For instance, one result of these internal conflicts would be the turning of aggression on oneself and resultant suicide-related behaviour.

Self-harm takes many forms and cutting is probably one that is very well known. It is difficult to gauge how many people cut themselves each year. For instance, in comparison to those who take overdoses, those who cut themselves are less likely to attend accident and emergency departments (Hawton *et al.*, 2002). More often than not the person will attend the accident and emergency department if they cut too deeply and require stitches. For instance, Lynn (1998, p. 36) states that she was scared when she cut too deeply and when blood squirted out. This suggests that her self-harm, albeit cutting, was not an attempt at suicide but that self-harm was a way to control feelings of helplessness and disempowerment. Other authors also suggest that cutting is frequently used by the person as a survival or coping strategy rather than as a destructive behaviour (Pembroke, 1998a, 1998b, 1998c ; Murphy, 2006; Zest, 2006). Also, while it is obvious that razor blades and knives would feature among the instruments used, it seems that any available instrument can be used to cut oneself. For example, at a conference in Derry City (Northern Ireland) in October 2003, one of the speakers told of how she used a blunt compass to cut herself (Zest, 2003). Most people would associate cutting with the person's wrists. However, frequently the person does not wish others to know of their self-harming behaviour and they will go out of their way to conceal it. For this reason, some people who self-harm may cut themselves on a part of their body that is generally hidden from public view. For example, and by no means exclusively, the abdomen, upper arms and legs are frequently used and some females cut themselves under their breasts. The reasons why a person may choose cutting as opposed to some other form of self-harm is not always obvious. For example, Lynn (1998) did not know why she started to cut herself. However, when she became depressed she resorted to cutting herself again and instantly felt better. She also went on to burn herself and because she felt good about it, the behaviour became an addiction for her. In addition, the National Institute for Clinical Excellence (NICE, 2004a) acknowledges that self-harm can happen in a way that is beyond a person's control and that some people do so whilst in a 'trance like' or dissociative state. When a person has no prospect of escape from a traumatic situation, then dissociation is a very common response. What happens is that the person does not feel real and feels that they have become disconnected from their real self. Bradshaw (1996, p. 129) calls it 'instant numbing' and states that 'the violence is so intolerable that the victim leaves his or her body'. This can be quite frightening for the person and one way of recon-necting themself with their true self is to injure themself. They can control the pain and this makes them feel real.

An early publication by Pembroke (1998b) makes the point that many females cut themselves and also that cutting is no respecter of any age group. However, in recent years, Hawton *et al.* (2004) have reported that those who cut themselves were more likely to be male, have a history of previous self-harm, live alone, misuse alcohol and have low suicide intent scores. Indeed, a recent consultation document in Northern Ireland (DHSSPSNI, 2006) states that recorded hospital admissions for self-harm is highest in both sexes in the 35–44-year-old age group but it is rare in those aged 75 years of age and over. In addition, Marchetto (2006) found no gender differences in people who choose to cut them-selves. Thus, it seems that cutting as a method of self-harm is used by both sexes and by people in different age groups.

Frequently, practitioners refer to self-harm as 'a cry for help'. Sometimes other practitioners refer to it as 'attention-seeking'. Both of these suggest that the person is trying to attract help or attention from others. Indeed, many practitioners would agree that the person is using self-harm, either consciously or uncon-sciously, as some form of social communication. Some would say that it is a 'cry for help'. Unfortunately, the combination of no suicidal intention and the 'cry for help' or 'attention-seeking' perception has in the past resulted in medical and nursing staff having negative attitudes to persons who self-harm (Ramon, Bancroft and Skrimshire, 1975; Patel, 1975; Hawton, Marsack and Fagg, 1981; Platt and Salter, 1987; Anon., 1990; Dunleavey, 1992). Also, physicians and nurses label those who self-harm as 'attention-seekers' (Platt and Salter, 1987). However, other researchers have found that casualty nurses (McLaughlin, 1994) and mental health nurses (Long and Reid, 1996) have more positive attitudes. Practitioners should not make assumptions about clients by using terms such as a 'cry for help' or 'attention-seeking'. Rather than place negative labels onto self-harm, practitioners should be more concerned about why the person is self-harming as it is an indicator of emotional despair in a fellow human being.

Thus, there are implications for how practitioners carry out their assessment of the person's psychological and emotional needs. Therefore, it is very important that health carers are thorough in their assessment. Unfortunately, when a person who self-harms is admitted to a statutory mental health facility, most practitioners will assume that the person is in a safe place and that their self-harming behaviour can be controlled. In reality it is the person who has control and it is the person who is self-harming who has the right to allow practitioners to intervene if required. It is incumbent on practitioners to establish a relationship with the person in order to understand them and why they choose to self-harm.

Repetitive self-harm

When self-harm is considered by practitioners it seems that what they are really referring to is repetitive self-harm. As mentioned earlier there is a very real possibility that many people who, on their first admission to hospital, are recorded as self-harming would in fact be more appropriately recorded as having attempted suicide. There is very little, if any, empirical literature to support the use of this latter statement. On the other hand, the current absence of any record of a person's intention at the time of the suicide-related behaviour does little to disprove this statement. Self-harm by definition does not indicate a wish or intention to die but it is quite possible that many of those who die as a result of their self-harming behaviour actually die by accident. It would be very inappropriate to call these self-harm-related deaths, it might be more appropriate to call these accidental deaths. Nevertheless, there is a risk of repeated self-harm in the three months following the initial behaviour (Hawton, 1991) and repetition rates of between 12% and 16% have been reported (Sakinofsky et al., 1990; Owens et al.,1994; Hawton et al., 2000). In recent times, some researchers have reported that approx 24% of persons repeat self-harm and there is very little difference between the proportion of males and females (Zahl and Hawton, 2004). Therefore, it would seem that at worst, some 75% of first presentations will not repeat the behaviour. Whether or not those 75% attempt suicide or self-harm at some stage in the future is a question that cannot be answered at this moment. Nonetheless, it is an intriguing question because it means that many of those who attend the accident and emergency department will not repeat the behaviour. Quite possibly, as in Case vignette 4 (Stephen), many of these may have been glad to survive and be able to review their options. In trying to find out the prevalence of those who repeat self-harm, practitioners are dependent on records maintained by local accident and emergency departments. Unfortunately, as discussed in Chapter 3, there are difficulties in the terminology and also in the coding of this behaviour. In addition, Lynn (1998) and Pembroke (1998a, 1998b) make the point that attending accident and emergency departments can be a harrowing experience for those who self-harm and for these reasons one attendance may be enough to drive the behaviour underground. One result of this is that the person will only attend the accident and emergency department when they really have to, and not because they want to.

However, those who repeat suicide-related behaviour seem to be character-ized by persistent interpersonal conflict (Kreitman and Casey, 1988). In addition, if a person is classified as having a personality disorder, then this will increase their chances of a repetition of suicide-related behaviour (Hawton, 1991). The risk of eventual suicide in those who repeat suicide-related behaviour is high (Rygnes-tad, 1988; Hawton, 1991; Gunnell et al., 1995; Johnsson Fridell, Ojehagen and Traskman-Bendz, 1996; Zahl and Hawton, 2004; Owens, Horrocks and House, 2002; Runeson, 2002; Cooper et al., 2005). For instance it is known that up to 50% of those people who die by suicide frequently have a history of a preceding suicide-related behaviour and many have been treated by their GP a short period before the fatal action (Kreitman, 1989). In addition, the risk of eventual suicide is higher if individuals take alcohol or abuse drugs (Hawton and Catalan, 1987; Hawton, 1994a). Therefore, a person who self-harms is at risk and any suicide-related behaviour that is referred to as 'attention-seeking' or a 'cry for help' requires serious consideration by practitioners.

Many of those who repetitively self-harm go to great lengths to conceal their suicide-related behaviour. Indeed, it seems that they are not looking for help or attention from others including health care practitioners. Nonetheless, if practi-tioners wish to help those who repetitively self-harm, then they need to review the way they deliver care and also change their perceptions of these people. For example, many practitioners focus their attention on the person's behaviour and try to stop the person self-harming by keeping the person safe and under constant observation. Unfortunately, this is not realistic in all cases as there is a person behind the behaviour. If practitioners focus only on the behaviour, then it is very likely that they will miss getting to know the real person and why they self-harm. How a person is feeling at the time they are self-harming is more important than the behaviour itself. Why is this? Well, self-harm is a form of therapy for many of those who choose it. It is their support system. They have, or believe that they have, control over their behaviour. Whether practitioners believe it or not it is the person who is self-harming that is expert in the behaviour. It is not their intention to die; in fact it is their intention to live. For instance, Pembroke (1998a) makes it very clear that if she could not have self-harmed, she wouldn't be here today.

In addition, the National Institute for Clinical Excellence (NICE, 2004a) also suggests that the purpose of self-harm is to preserve life. Unfortunately, some practitioners feel that they have to intervene, as they believe that the person is at risk of suicide. Maybe now is a time for practitioners to review their beliefs about self-harm and instead make efforts to try understanding why the person has self-harmed.

Summary

The focus in this chapter was on the concept of suicide-related behaviour and exploring each of the components within it. The assertion made here is that all forms of suicide-related behaviour can end in the death of a person. However, inherent within suicide-related behaviour are both life and death components. The death component is attempted suicide. Where there is evidence that the person tried to kill him or herself, then practitioners must acknowledge it. In so doing they will acknowledge the emotional pain and the psychache of the person. The use of other terms, other than attempted suicide, could result in practitioners making different interpretations and this may impact on the type of care required by the person. Ambivalence is frequently linked to suicide-related behaviour. While ambivalence contains both death and life components, there is danger until the person makes a decision to grasp the life component. Also, it is asserted here that ambivalence in a person is above the non-zero level of suicide intent and therefore any form of suicide-related behaviour must be treated as attempted suicide.

In contrast, suicide-related behaviour also includes a life component. The life component is self-harm. In self-harm the person's intention is not to die but to obtain relief of some emotional pain or psychache. In a way their self-harm, while being personal and secretive to them, is also a communication to others. They are looking for help. However, many of those who self-harm do not seek help from practitioners. For instance, the literature suggests that some practitioners have negative attitudes to those who self-harm. Sometimes there is a stigma attached or the fear of being diagnosed as being mentally ill. If practitioners are ever going to gain the confidence of people who self-harm, then they must review their attitudes and their care strategies towards those who self-harm.

Repetitive self-harm is probably the suicide-related behaviour that creates most difficulty for practitioners. Certainly, the literature makes it clear that negative attitudes do exist towards those who are repetitively admitted. It seems that some practitioners focus their attention on the person's self-harming behaviour. The literature suggests that the focus may be better spent on focusing on the person. Certainly, the viewpoint that is emphasized here is that it is understanding the person that is important. Once that is achieved then practitioners can move with the person to make efforts to resolve the issues that cause them emotional pain.

In Chapter 5 the focus is on the various ways that a person can descend into crisis and come to the point where suicide-related behaviour becomes an option.

The descent into crisis

5

In Chapter 5 the following issues are explored:

1. Why suicide-related behaviour?
2. What are stressors?
3. Theoretical perspectives on stressors
   (a) The biological perspective
   (b) The psychological perspective
   (c) The psychoanalytical perspective
   (d) The psychodynamic developmental perspective
   (e) The cognitive perspective
   (f) The situational or stressful life events perspective
   (g) The social integration perspective
   (h) The mental ill-health perspective
4. Crisis

Why suicide-related behaviour?

Why do people want to kill themselves? Why do people kill themselves? Why do people self-harm? Family, friends and even practitioners frequently ask these questions. There is no one specific answer to any of these questions. The reasons for this are that there are many causes and life events that can lead a person to consider suicide-related behaviour. In trying to understand why a person chooses to kill him or herself or to self-harm depends very much on practitioners' attitudes towards the person and their efforts to communicate with the person. In addition, it can also depend very much on the person's willingness to communicate with practitioners. The reality is that the person knows why they have chosen a suicide-related behaviour, whereas practitioners can but estimate from the information obtained from assessments. What we do know is that most incidences of suicide-related behaviour are preceded by very stressful events. For instance, Paykel, Prusoff and Myers (1975) found that those persons who attempted suicide had almost four times as many negative life events as those in the general population. Whether or not a person in crisis chooses self-harm, attempts suicide or dies as a result of suicide depends on a number of events. In this chapter, Figure 5.1 outlines a potential pathway that a person may have taken on their journey towards crisis and the possibility of suicide-related behaviour. In this pathway, the descent into crisis and the darkness of self-harm and suicide can begin with a number of causes. The academic literature indicates that external incidences or events that create distress in the person are the same as those that can lead to despair and future suicide-related behaviour. These incidents are frequently called stressors.

It is well known that the onset of stress in a person can lead to positive responses in both the way a person thinks and also how they behave. This type of stress is frequently called Eustress. However, it is also well known that stress can have negative effects on the way a person thinks and behaves. This negative type of stress can lead to distress in the person. Frequently, distress, despair and resultant crisis are precursors of suicide-related behaviour. When considering the origins of suicide-related behaviour there are a number of theoretical perspectives, which can offer both rationale for the behaviour and potential caring and therapeutic responses. Such perspectives include biological, psychological, sociological and situational. In addition, quite a number of research-based articles suggest that self-harm and suicide can come from any one of a set of risk factors. Many of these risk factors have been identified from research reports that focused on those who engaged in and survived either self-harm or attempted suicide.

It must be made clear that no one theoretical or other viewpoint can offer a stand-alone explanation for either self-harm or attempted suicide. Frequently, one theoretical perspective may offer an explanation for self-harm and attempted suicide. For example, the situational perspective offers a sometimes too simplistic here-and-now basis for the development of distress within the person. This perspective may be right on a number of occasions. However, the clever or astute practitioner will ensure that other possible perspectives are explored while assessing the person's mental health care needs. This will make sure that an accurate depiction of the person's intentions is gained. While Figure 5.1 outlines a potential pathway towards self-harm and attempted suicide, it is in

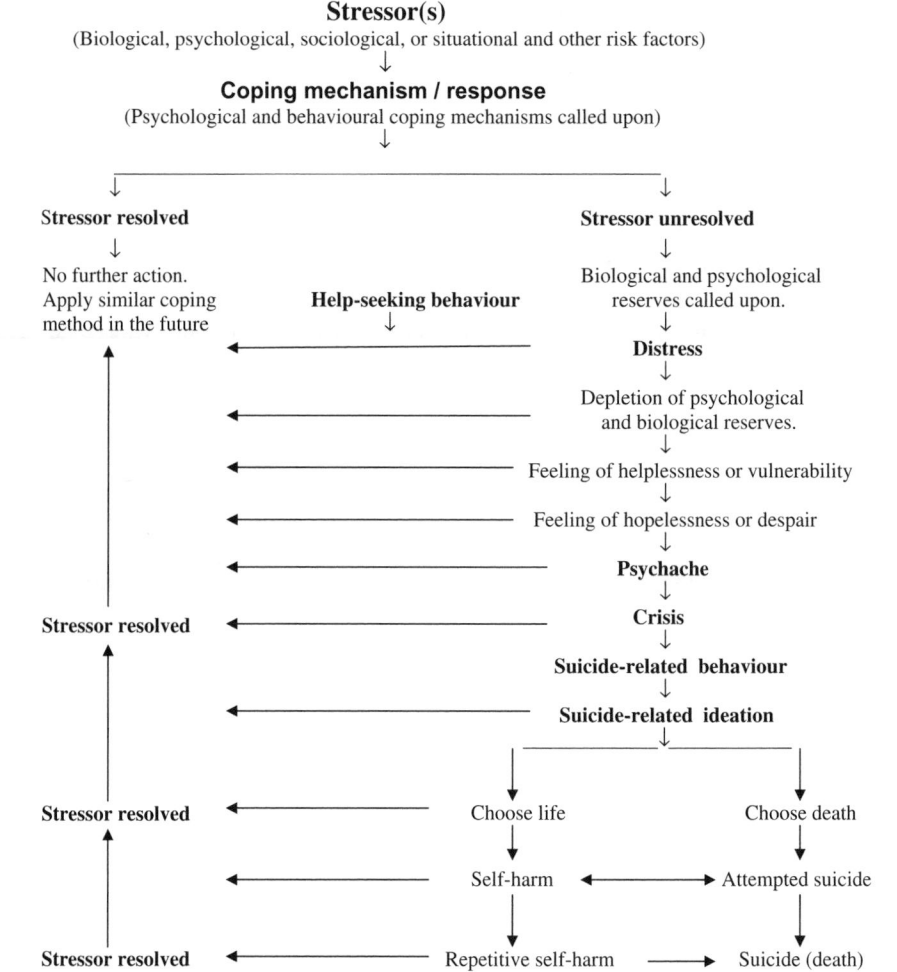

Fig. 5.1 A pathway towards crisis and suicide-related behaviour.

reality a summary of my current thinking. At this point in time Figure 5.1 can remind the practitioner of the potential journey that a person may have taken prior to seeking and obtaining help. I am confident that some students will find Figure 5.1 useful but I have no doubt that in the future other more learned researchers may critically analyse and more accurately define each of the steps that lead a person into crisis and then into the darkness of suicide-related behaviour.

What are stressors?

In brief, a stressor is a situation that arises or an event that occurs and places a physical or psychological demand on the person. Most authors would agree that in general, there are a number of theoretical perspectives where stressors can evolve. These are:

- **Biological perspective:** Infections, physical injury/trauma, disease, thirst, malnutrition, and fatigue. However, much of the current research focuses on the belief that low levels of neurotransmitters such as serotonin or norepinephrine at the nerve synapses are major contributors in the development of suicide-related behaviour.

- **Psychological perspective:** The threat of physical harm, attacks or the threat of attacks on the person's self esteem or belief system, guilt or the thought of impending doom are examples of psychological stressors. Other more generalized psychological perspectives are: the psychoanalytical perspective, the psychodynamic developmental perspective, and the cognitive perspective.

- **Sociological perspective:** Much of the research in this perspective focuses on how integrated the person is into society. For example, the person's social networks and particularly the lack of social networks can underpin a person's suicidal thoughts.

- **Situational:** These tend to be very specific stressors and relate to major events that occur in the person's life. These events can be very stress inducing. For example, exam stress, economic pressure, bullying, loss of a job, poor housing, overcrowding, difficulties in interpersonal relationships or the break-up of a relationship and the death of a partner.

However, while there are numerous types of stressors, what may be a stressor to one person may have little or very little impact on another. Also, if the same stressor impacts on two or more people at the same time, each person may react to it quite differently. Being very much social beings, people are constantly exposed to stressors in their lives. For example, any of the following may cause distress in people: physical illness; bullying at school; abuse (sexual, physical, or emotional); seeking a job; relationship difficulties; marriage; divorce; death of a partner, friend or family member; moving house; and ageing. These are just a few but the list is endless. While a single stressor can impinge on the person's well-being, Lazarus (1981) warns that too many daily 'hassles' can also overwhelm the person. However, providing the stressor is not too severe and that stressors do not accumulate, most people are quite capable of coping with many of the stressors they meet during the course of any day. Many people who have been confronted with excessive stressors usually, in time, work things out and get on with their lives. In contrast, other people find it difficult to cope with even small amounts of stress or minor stressors and if relief is not found these can lead to feelings of vulnerability or despair and possibly suicide-related behaviour.

Some people bear the scars of long-lasting psychological trauma. More often than not this is due to the type and the number of stressors that occur in their lives. When a person is faced with excessive external demands, his or her normal coping mechanisms may fail and (s)he may resort to ineffective or inappropriate behaviours to try and resolve them. This behavioural reaction could result in physical illness and psychological symptoms such as anxiety, depression or panic. In an effort to release some of the tension within themselves, the person may even become violent towards others. At the very extreme, their violence may be turned against themselves and it may result in permanent physical damage to their body or even in extreme cases it may result in the person's death or the death of others whether by intention or accident.

No matter what the stressor is, most people will try to resolve the incident that is causing the stress. They will try to adjust their lives or compensate in some other way to reduce the physical and psychological effects of the stressor. If a person's coping methods are successful and the stressor is overcome, the matter will be resolved and the person will learn and usually adapt the same coping response to similar stressors in the future. For example, earlier I summarized Mark's story in Case vignette 22. About a year after our last therapeutic engagement, Mark called to see me again. At this meeting he told me of the progress in his life and in his business after successfully regaining his driving licence. In addition, he explained how he used our role-play scenarios to heal a rift between one of his siblings and his parents. He applied the same principles that we used during our sessions. Thus, as indicated in Figure 5.1, it is possible even when a person is considering suicide that difficulties can be resolved, stressors and their effects can be overcome and the person can learn and adapt their behaviour. This learning can in turn be used in the future if crisis arises again.

However, if the person's coping efforts are unsuccessful and the effects of the stressor worsen, the person may feel that they can do no more, have nowhere else to go to or no one to turn to. At this point the person, just like Mark, will experience crisis. Depending on the person's thinking at the time, (s)he may play one last (presumably) trump card in an effort to resolve the crisis. If this fails, (s)he may then choose other maladaptive behaviours to lessen the emotional pain. While any form of behavioural response could be encountered, these behaviours could include the options of self-harm or suicide.

Theoretical perspectives on stressors

This section explores some of the more common theoretical perspectives that underpin the understanding of stressors and how they lead to self-harm and suicide. In each perspective there are clues as to the type of therapy that might be useful in resolving or reducing the effects of the stressor. In brief, the perspectives are: biological, psychological (psychoanalytical, psychodynamic developmental, cognitive theory, situational or stressful life changes theory), and the sociological perspective (social integration theory).

(a) The biological perspective

The biological perspective was for a number of years the primary model used by a number of practitioners in the medical and allied professions to assess and treat persons who contemplate suicide-related behaviour. For instance, it has long been thought that there is a link between a malfunction in the biochemistry of the brain and suicide-related behaviour. In brief, it is suggested that it is this malfunction in the biochemistry of the brain that leads a person to consider and carry out some form of suicide-related behaviour. Much of the research that has studied the biochemical links to suicide-related behaviour has focused on estimating the levels of several neurotransmitters in the synapses. Some of these neurotransmitters are serotonin (5-hydroxytryptamine or also called 5-HT); dopamine; lithium and norepinephrine. Among these, the neurotransmitter serotonin, which affects mood and emotions, appears to have some prominence. In this section, by focusing on the research on serotonin, it will be possible to consider both the positive and negative aspects of the biological perspective that could lead towards suicide-related behaviour.

In a study of cerebro-spinal fluid (CSF) metabolites, van Praag *et al.* (1970) reported a correlation between low levels of a metabolite called 5-hyroxyindoleacetic acid (5-HIAA) and depression. 5-HIAA is produced when the neurotransmitter serotonin is broken down in the body. Thus, 5-HIAA is a waste product of serotonin. A few years later, Ashberg, Traskman and Thoren (1976) reported that significantly more depressed persons in the low CSF 5-HIAA group had a history of attempted suicide-related behaviour than those persons in the high CSF 5-HIAA group. The suggestion here was that a low level of the metabolite 5-HIAA indicates a low level of serotonin and this in turn may stimulate suicide-related behaviour in such people. One follow-up study of people who had attempted suicide found that low levels of 5-HIAA predicted those who would attempt suicide within the next five years (Roy, DeJong and Linnoila, 1989). The work by these researchers suggested that low levels of the metabolite 5-HIAA could act as a possible suicide predictor.

Other researchers made advances in the study of serotonin and its relationship with suicide-related behaviour. For example, Nordstrom *et al.* (1994) used lumbar puncture to determine levels of 5-HIAA in a sample of persons (n = 92) admitted following attempted suicide. Almost 12% of these persons killed themselves within one year and eight of these had low levels of CSF 5-HIAA metabolites. Nonetheless, what was also noticed was that over an average of six years of observation some 85% of the sample did not die by suicide. Secondly, Verkes *et al.* (1996) measured blood platelet levels of serotonin (5-HT) and monoamine oxidase-B in a sample of 54 people who repetitively attempted suicide. They came to the conclusion that low serotonin could apply to recurrent suicide attempters. A main limitation with Verkes *et al.*'s (1996) work was the lack of an appropriate 'control' group. Also, Muck-Seler, Jakovljevic and Pivac (1996) examined the levels of platelet 5-HT in the blood and found that there were different platelet 5-HT concentrations in psychotic and non-psychotic depressed persons. This finding led to the presumption that there was a subtype of depression that was biologically distinct. They also found that the most violent forms of suicide-related behaviour were associated with the lowest platelet 5-HT concentrations.

However, while it could be assumed that low serotonin was linked only to depression, it is interesting to note that similar links were found in persons with other psychiatric diagnoses. For example, van Praag (1983) found low levels of CSF 5-HIAA in non-depressed persons diagnosed with schizophrenia. In addition, other authors reported that there were links between low CSF 5-HIAA and increased levels of outward-directed aggression in those with personality disorder (Brown *et al.*, 1979; Coccaro, 1992). This link was stronger when the aggressive behaviour was of an impulsive nature (Cremniter *et al.*, 1999). Similarly, it was reported that there were associations between low CSF 5-HIAA and aggressive behaviour in non-human research (Higley *et al.*, 1993; Mehlmann *et al.*, 1994). These findings suggest that while low serotonin is associated with depression and suicide-related behaviour, it seems to be very much more associated with mood disturbance and particularly with aggressive behaviour. These findings may thus give rationale as to why people direct aggression inward towards the self and on other occasions outward towards others.

In more recent times van Praag (2001, p. 70) has proposed that the link between dysfunction in the serotonergic system and suicide-related behaviour may not be purely biological. While maintaining that dysfunctions in the serotonergic system are associated with a destabilization of the regulation of anxiety and aggression, van Praag (2001) also asserted that when stress is sustained it can lead to cortisol overproduction and this can provoke or aggravate serotonergic disturbances. These assertions have led van Praag (2001, pp. 70–1) to hypothesize that dysfunctions in the levels of serotonin are 'biological characteristics that increase the risk of suicide in times of mounting stress and thus can be regarded as biological risk factors for suicide-related behaviour'. However, this hypothesis requires testing.

There are a number of reasons why care must be taken in analysing or depending too heavily on biological results. First, lumbar puncture is an aseptic invasive procedure involving the insertion of a needle into the lumbar spinal sac and withdrawing a sample of CSF for analysis. Therefore, it is not without complications. Second, the levels of CSF 5-HIAA do not give an accurate indication of serotonin levels in the brain. Third, Molcho, Stanley and Stanley (1991) reported conflicting evidence regarding post-mortem levels of 5-HIAA in the brains of suicide victims. Fourth, in Nordstrom *et al.* (1994), the range of values may produce a large number of 'false positives'. For example, 85% of their sample did not kill themselves. Fifth, there are many factors affecting CSF concentrations of 5-HIAA (sex, height, age, drug treatment and diet are but a few). Sixth, there is scepticism concerning accepting biological factors as sole precursors to serious mental illness (Dawson, 1997) and similar arguments could apply to research on suicide-related behaviour (van Praag, 2001). Seventh, the low predictability has to be balanced against the expense of large-scale testing in a time of scarce health care resources. Therefore, practitioners and researchers need to be careful before suggesting that the biological perspective can predict future suicide or suicide-related behaviour in all cases.

These findings contribute to the debate on both the aetiology and the predictability of suicide but at this point in time it would be premature to accept that there is a sole biological marker for suicide-related behaviour. However, the research into the possible links between human biology and suicide-related behaviour gives a sense that in the future it may have a predictive value in some cases. For example, the studies of Verkes *et al.* (1996) and Muck-Seler, Jakovljevic and Pivac (1996) suggest that in the future it may be possible to identify those at risk of suicide by examining serotonin levels through routine blood samples. However, until this becomes common practice in the future, all practitioners would need to take cognisance of the limitations of a purely biological perspective.

(b) The psychological perspective

This perspective adds to the knowledge portrayed in the biological perspective. However, while the biological perspective offers mainly a medical approach, the psychological perspective offers a much broader theoretical base from which self-harm and suicide may stem. Links between emotional and psychological difficulties and suicidal ideation, self-harm and attempted suicide are well known (Hawton and Fagg, 1992; Hawton *et al.*, 2000; Lawlor and James, 2000). Therefore, considering perspectives that focus on the person's cognitive and behavioural development will give practitioners a broader foundation in trying to understand how psychological stressors can lead to self-harm and suicide.

(c) The psychoanalytical perspective

Sigmund Freud was the creator of psychoanalytic theory. His writings extend from his first publication *The Interpretation of Dreams* (1900) to his final manuscript *An Outline of Psychoanalysis* (1940). For this reason, only a brief outline of relevant aspects of Freud's psychoanalytical theory can be presented here. In psychoanalytic theory the basic philosophy is that development in human beings is very much determined by the person's experiences in childhood. For example, psychoanalytic theory asserts that personality difficulties in adulthood are attributed to repressed childhood conflicts. Also, the person's behaviour is influenced by unconscious motives and conflicts and also by aggressive and sexual impulses. In addition, the development of a normal personality is based very much on the child's successful resolution and assimilation of the psychosexual stages in childhood development. Therefore, if the child fails to resolve any of these psychosexual stages adequately then faulty personality development will be the result. Furthermore, in psychoanalytic theory, the personality is made up of three parts:

1. The id is the unconscious part that consists of basic instincts such as sexual and aggressive impulses. The sexual part is also called libido. The id is with the child practically from birth. It seeks immediate gratification.

2. The ego is the rational and conscious part of the personality and it develops at about two years of age. The ego operates on the reality principle. The ego weighs up the selfishness of the id with the morals of the super-ego and will act accordingly. It's the ego that suffers when wrong decisions are taken.

3. The super-ego is formed when the child is about five years of age and is very much influenced by parental, social and religious morals. The super-ego is partially conscious and also partially unconscious. The conscious part of the super-ego is formed when the child is punished and is made to feel guilty for misbehaving. However, the ego-ideal part is developed when the child behaves appropriately and is rewarded for doing so.

More often than not, the three parts of the personality are in conflict. These conflicts are frequently between the id, which wants it basic instincts satisfied now, and the super-ego, which will look to maintain moral standards. The ego tries to balance the conflicts between the id and the super-ego and this can give rise to difficulties.

When conflicts between the id and the super-ego take place, anxiety can arise in the person. In order to control this anxiety the ego can call upon the mental defence mechanisms of which a number are well known such as: projection, denial, repression, reaction formation, displacement, regression, rationalization, and sublimation. For instance, when something goes wrong for a person, in order to protect their own integrity they might blame others. This is called projection. These defence mechanisms are very powerful and they operate by protecting the person from any anxiety that may arise as a result of their own behaviour or their inability to deal with the behaviour of others. For instance, the person may deny that a traumatic event such as bereavement has occurred. Another example, displacement, is where a person may feel angry at work and they go home and take their emotions out on their family. However, repression is where a person has suffered a traumatic event and rather than deal with the issues or because they cannot at that time deal with the issues, they keep the memory of the event out of consciousness. The astute student will notice that repressed memories in a person's mind have the potential to come back into consciousness and create difficulties in later life.

One early trend in psychoanalytic thinking was to link Freud's (1917/1957) theory of melancholia with the dynamics of depression (Meissner, 1977). This model emphasizes the internalization of a lost, ambivalently loved object, resulting in self-devaluation and self-destructive behaviour (Lovett and Maltsberger, 1992). Freud (1922/1984) distinguishes between the life instincts (or Eros) including sexuality, and the death instincts (or Thanatos) including aggression. In addition, these instincts are influenced by the triumvirate theory of personality involving the id, the ego, and the super-ego. Freud attempted to explain suicide-related behaviour in terms of internal conflicts between the demands of the id on one hand, and the demands of the super-ego and reality on the other. One result of these internal conflicts is the turning of aggression towards the self, with resultant self-harm or actual suicide.

As mentioned earlier, psychoanalytical theory concentrates on childhood experiences as determinants of adult behaviour and experience. For example, Leonard (1967, p. 313) suggests 'that the seeds for future suicidal potential are sown in the second and third years of life'. In this stage, which equates with Freud's (1905/1977) 'anal stage', crucial experiences occur that set the child's ensuing developmental pattern in a rigid mould, which leaves him vulnerable in later life to suicide-related behaviour, given specific environmental pressures (Leonard, 1967). Failure to achieve may cause the child to doubt his or her present abilities and has implications when facing challenges in later life. A key belief within psychoanalytical theory is that faulty personality traits develop as a result of the child not being able to resolve, or that the child inadequately resolves, issues at some particular stage in childhood. Other researchers have noted a sequential pattern of interpersonal difficulty from early childhood (Silove, George and Bhavani-Sankaram, 1987; McLeod, 1991; Carrigan, 1994; Evans, 1994). These findings give additional support to Freud's theory and suggest that childhood experiences require exploration, as do those suicides and attempted suicides that are reported in children (Hawton, 1982; Brookshank, 1985; Friedman and Corn, 1985; McLaughlin and Whittington, 1996).

Freud is often thought of as the Father of Psychoanalysis. His views are that talking about personal issues that cause psychache is the basis for most of the counselling approaches used today. His talk therapy methodology was a combination of 'free association' and 'catharsis'. In order to bring adults' inner conflicts into the open, and to seek resolution of these conflicts, these early childhood experiences are explored in therapy. If the person in therapy is able to release repressed feelings associated with the conflict, the symptoms should recede. In the UK, Evans (1994) gives an in-depth account of the practical use of psychoanalytic theory as an approach to the care of the suicidal person. However, although there is support for psychoanalytical theory, it remains outside the broad canon of scientifically orientated mental health practice. It is also limited by its emphasis upon the explanatory power of childhood events and experiences. Despite that, it has made an important contribution to our understanding of how self-harm and suicide occur and to possible therapeutic interventions.

(d) The psychodynamic developmental perspective

Erikson (1977) described the 'Eight Ages of Man', each of which presents the person with a new developmental task to be achieved. This expanded on Freud's work by considering development throughout the lifespan, rather than focusing only on childhood development. For example, in Erikson's (1977) 'Autonomy versus Shame and Doubt Stage' children try to be autonomous. Failure to achieve successfully at this stage may cause children to doubt their ability to become autonomous and these doubts can have implications when facing challenges in later life. In addition, children can learn to feel guilty about their behaviour. If this behaviour does not match up to another person's ideals then the child may feel shame and could feel humiliated as well. The development of shame or of being humiliated may increase the intensity of emotional turmoil in adolescence or adulthood. Indeed, Shea (2002) makes the point that shame and humiliation are probably the most common driving force towards suicide-related behaviour among adolescents. In the 'Identity Versus Role Confusion' stage, which occurs during adolescence, teenagers can face an identity crisis and an unsuccessful outcome can result in identity confusion (Erikson, 1977, 1985). In Northern Ireland, McLaughlin and Whittington (1996) reported a high incidence of suicide per se in the 15–24-year-old age group and the wider academic and research-based literature abounds with examples of self-harm and attempted suicides for the same group (Catalan, 1983; Shaffer *et al.*, 1988; Remafedi, Farrow and Deisher,

1991; Andrus *et al.*, 1991; Hawton and Fagg, 1992; Champion, Goodall and Rutter, 1995; Schmidtke *et al.*, 1996; Hawton *et al.*, 2000).

Many of life's difficulties can and frequently do arise in childhood. For instance, many children are taught to obey others in authority such as parents, church leaders and teachers. It is very normal for children to explore their world and to experiment with what they are allowed to do. Children must learn to conform to society and to adhere to society's codes. However, how parents and other influential adults impose these social and moral codes on children could affect the child in later life. For instance, what effect will criticism, hostility or ridicule have on the emotional and cognitive development of a child? If they do not learn properly at school they may be made to feel stupid by others such as classmates, teachers and parents. If a child breaks religious codes they may feel guilt or shame. More often than not destructive criticism by others can lead people, of any age, to feel inadequate and unable to cope with life's difficulties. However, Erikson's theory covers more than childhood and adolescent development. The theory also extends into old age in the 'Integrity versus Despair' stage. In this stage, the person reflects back on their life and in the integrity part they seek assurances that their lives have been meaningful, that they have achieved and are now ready to face old age and death at some stage. However, they can feel despair if in their evaluation they see only failures or a life with a number of unaccomplished goals.

Erikson's theory has made a valuable contribution to the understanding of self-harm and suicide by suggesting stages where crises can occur during the lifespan. Implicit in these views is the need for a clinical method of assessing a person's development throughout the lifespan and identifying the origins of psychological crises. Peplau (1952) was the first to coin the phrase nurse–patient relationship and her theory of mental health nursing was based on psychodynamic principles. In applying the principles of psychodynamic developmental theory Fitzpatrick *et al.* (1982) suggested that practitioners should focus on the person's current level of development and the interaction between the id, ego, and super-ego. The main aim of therapy would be to resolve the conflict between the person's id (selfish and basic) impulses and their super-ego (moralistic selves) and then assist the person to progress through to the next stage of their development. However, the link between psychoanalytic theory and psychodynamic developmental theory should not be ignored, as difficulties in earlier life do resurrect themselves in later life and can create emotional difficulties for the person (Evans, 1994). Some of these can include feelings of shame and possibly humiliation. Also, the person may have poor coping mechanisms and may find it difficult to resolve emotional issues or express their emotions. Certainly, some researchers have found that in counselling sessions male adolescents consider that being able to talk about their emotions was more important than the cognitive categories (Dunne *et al.*, 2000). Also, other researchers have reported similar results in adults (Cummings, Slemon and Hallberg, 1993; Elliott and Wexler, 1994). While the psychodynamic developmental perspective suggests how and where difficulties can arise in person, it is very much implicit that any assessment of the person's emotional needs should explore each stage of their development.

(e) The cognitive perspective

Cognitive theory suggests that life's experiences lead people to form functional or dysfunctional assumptions about themselves. These assumptions structure how a person perceives him or herself and they can influence the person's evaluation of their performance in any behaviour. For example, if a person's behaviour results in a successful outcome, then evaluation of the self and the behaviour is likely to be positive and the behaviour is likely to be repeated in the future. Therefore, learning from previous experience is a principal component of cognitive theory. The clinical application of cognitive theory is 'Cognitive Therapy' and a person's difficulties are viewed as emanating from distorted thinking (cognition) that is learned and is self-defeating (Russell and Morrill, 1989). To address distorted cognitions, Mahoney (1974) and Meichenbaum (1977) emphasize cognitive restructuring to change maladaptive learning.

Cognitive theory lends itself to explanations of positive evaluations of the self and behaviour, but the reverse is also possible. For instance, depression is characterized by negative thoughts (Haaga, Dyck and Ernst, 1991). Secondly, there is evidence that failing to cope with stressful life events can result in self-harm and in attempted suicide (Farmer and Creed, 1989; Nordentoft and Rubin, 1993; Gould et al., 1996). Thirdly, cognitive distortion is a predictor of suicidal intent (Mendonca and Holden, 1996). Repetitive failure and resultant negative cognitions can lead to learned self-helplessness (Seligman, 1975), hopelessness or pessimism about the future (Beck, Kovacs and Weissman, 1975; Beck et al., 1979; Bolland, 2003), and eventual self-harm or attempted suicide (Beck, Kovacs and Weissman, 1975; Beck et al., 1993; Shneidman, 1992; MacLeod, Rose and Williams, 1993; Morano, Cisler and Lemerond, 1993). In brief, when a person's behaviour fails to resolve an event or incident that induces stress, then the person may develop dysfunctional assumptions about themselves and these assumptions may become rigid.

Dysfunctional assumptions can arise not only from previous behaviour, but they can also arise from beliefs about the self. For example, it is not uncommon for the media and teenage magazines to report that many adolescent females perceive themselves as being ugly and have a negative body image of themselves. Also, some people assume that other people see them as useless; therefore after a period of time they begin to think that they are useless. From wherever a person's negative cognition or dysfunctional assumptions arise, once activated, they can produce an upsurge of negative automatic thoughts (Mahoney, 1974; Fennell, 1989; Moorley, 1995; Sheldon, 1995). These thoughts are 'negative' as they are pessimistic and 'automatic' and they occur spontaneously. Usually these negative thoughts involve the past, current life experiences, or predictions about the future (Mahoney, 1974). In suicide-related behaviour, these automatic negative thoughts would create severe distress in the person. The person may feel so useless that they eventually lose hope for the future and the development of despair could result in the person contemplating or carrying out some form of suicide-related behaviour. For example, the suicide note left by Kurt Cobain suggests that he had very negative thoughts about himself. According to the suicide note, Kurt felt very guilty about the way he portrayed his feelings during performances and he did not want to fool his family, his fans or his band members. In addition, Kurt suffered for a long time with undiagnosed stomach pains. These pains were probably due to an ulcer. These pains caused him a lot of worry and exacerbated his negative thoughts of himself. He could no longer handle these negative thoughts and felt that suicide was the answer. It is quite clear that Kurt Cobain had had enough of the psychache or emotional pain and the physical pain that had been developing within him for a number of years.

Cognitive theory has made a significant contribution to the understanding and development of self-harm and attempted suicide in people by suggesting processes through which negative thoughts, depression, hopelessness and crisis can develop. Negative thoughts can, if not interrupted, lead to depression, which in turn increases their frequency. A vicious circle is created as the more depressed the person becomes, the more depressing thoughts they think, and the more they believe them. The circle can progress into a downward spiral towards crisis. The interruption of this circle is crucial if a person is to return to a more stable emotional and psychological state.

(f) The situational or stressful life events perspective

This perspective is different from previous perspectives as it refers mainly to the here and now and focuses on recent stressful events in a person's life. As mentioned earlier, most suicide-related behaviour is preceded by stressful life events (Paykel, Prusoff and Myers, 1975). More often than not, the stressor(s) is current and a person can frequently put a time and date on when the stressor impinged on their physical, emotional and psychological well-being. In brief, any specific life event or situation that is perceived by the person as an excessive demand or a threat may become the stressor. These stressors can include both positive (marriage celebrations) and negative (divorce proceedings) life events. The importance of considering such events has been highlighted in Gould et al. (1996) and in Hawton et al. (2000). In addition, stressful life events are very much related to self-harm (NICE, 2004a).

Early authors felt that stress lay in a particular relationship between the person and the situation (Lazarus and Folkman, 1984). Depending on the event the person will evaluate his abilities to meet the demands of the situation. If the situation is unimportant to the person and (s)he is unable to meet the demands of the situation, the person will more than likely not experience any stress. However, if the event is important enough to the person and in his or her evaluation they find that they cannot meet the demands then stress is very likely to occur. For example, earlier I mentioned a person called Mark (Case vignette 22) who was caught by the police, charged and convicted for drunken driving. In Mark's case, he had his own business, owned the vehicle, and needed his driving licence for his work. The loss of his driving licence was a big price to pay for his drunk-driving offence. In addition, the thought of telling his elderly parents about his impending conviction was also creating difficulty for him. Therefore, it is not surprising that his anxiety levels were at an all time high. In fairness to Mark, he accepted his punishment, got on with his life and no longer drinks and drives. Mark's anxiety came from a mixture of events that included having to tell his elderly parents about his impending conviction and also the impending loss of driving licence, an important thing in his working life. A key feature in Mark's suicidal feelings was the thought of the shame that his behaviour would bring on himself and his family. It is well known, particularly in Japanese culture, that public shame and humiliation or even the thought that it is going to happen could result in the ritual of *seppuku*. Stressors such as these may become exaggerated and the person may feel that they cannot prevent the possibility of public humiliation. In this situation the person may have catastrophic thoughts and sometimes it may seem that suicide-related behaviour is the only option available. How else does a person avert humiliation? However, another person in a similar situation may not exhibit the same anxiety levels. For whatever reasons, they may lack any feelings of guilt or shame. In addition, driving a car may not be too important to them as they probably could arrange lifts to work with friends.

Closely linked to the above example is the work of Snow *et al.* (2002) who highlighted the increasing trends in suicide in English and Welsh prisons. In addition, Snow (2002) also reported on prisoners' motives for all forms of suicide-related behaviour. One of the main motivational factors of suicide-related behaviour was concern about forthcoming court cases. These seem to relate very well with the shame and guilt of their behaviour and the possibility of being humiliated in court. For instance, the feelings that Mark (Case vignette 22) felt about the humiliation the court case would bring was enough for him to consider suicide. Thus, it seems that impending negative events, such as court appearances, can create distress in individuals and that this distress could lead a person to consider suicide-related behaviour as a way or dealing with the stressor.

Another example of a specific situation is that of bullying. While bullying in schools is a well-known and very worrying phenomenon, it is also acknowledged that bullying can involve adults and can occur in the workplace. In this book the main focus will be on bullying in childhood. For example, during 2005 in the United Kingdom, a number of children killed themselves as a result of bullying. These cases made national headlines in the media and schools were asked to review their policies on bullying. It is well known that bullying in schools is a major situational stressor and it must be acknowledged that it has happened to many people. In primary schools, bullying most often occurs in the playground where another classmate bullies females, and older boys bully males. However, in secondary schools older females most often bully females and boys are more likely to be bullied by classmates. Bullying need not be just physical, it can be mental as well and this is very difficult for the person who is bullied. Anyone can be bullied including television stars as well (Oddy, 2006). It is difficult to link bullying to self-harm or suicide. However, Father Brian D'Arcy, writing in the *Sunday World* (20 February 2005), believes that it is the root cause of many suicides in young children in Ireland. Bullying can take the form of mental and physical intimidation and social exclusion and can include aggression, name-calling, and spreading true or false rumours. All are very hurtful to the person being bullied and school holidays can come as a major relief to some. However, the return to school after a holiday period can be very difficult for pupils.

Let us consider that a definition of bullying could include the exertion of power and control over another person. Also, let us further consider that the bullied person would experience fear, intimidation, humiliation, depression, have feelings of isolation and a fear of reprisal. Additionally, that as a result of bullying, the person's own self-esteem would be systematically dismantled by the bully. These are the ingredients for future self-harm and suicide in the victim of bullying. For some pupils the bullying can be relentless and can lead to suicidal ideation and to self-harm (Mackinnon, 2005; MHF/CF, 2006). However, for other pupils bullying can end in suicide (Chapman, 2005).

Consider the following scenario from a child's point of view. What can a child do when (s)he is being bullied at school? Should they tell the teachers? Would this stop the bullying? Should the child tell his parents? Would they tell the teachers? Would this stop the bullying? Or would the bullying continue in a more secretive manner? For instance, consider the following:

1. Child reports bullying to teacher
2. Teacher reports bullying to head teacher
3. Head teacher has discussion with bully or bullies and pupils who are being bullied.
4. Bully promises to stop! Does this happen usually?

Most, if not all, schools currently have anti-bullying policies. How these policies are operated may differ between schools. Certainly there is evidence that having good policies does not mean that bullying is being effectively managed (Panorama, 2005). Nonetheless, in all cases there are three fundamental issues worth remembering: (1) the (bullied) student needs to feel safe, supported and that the bullying will cease, (2) the bully(s) must recognize that their behaviour is wrong and punishable (within child protection legislation), and (3) the bully(s) may need help themselves. In protecting vulnerable people who are being bullied, the most important issue is that appropriate action is taken to ensure that the bullying ceases. While there is evidence of good practice in some schools, it is unfortunate that appropriate action is not taken in all schools (Panorama, 2005). The impact that bullying has on schoolchildren cannot be underestimated as Rigby (2000) concluded that frequent peer victimization contributes significantly towards poor mental health in adolescents.

The stressful life events perspective suggests that stressors may take many forms in people and are very much dependent on the person's own personality traits, the importance they place on the event and their ability to deal effectively with any situation that arises. In general, the person's difficulty is frequently apparent; they can explain the nature of their difficulty but find it hard to deal with it. In an attempt to measure the impact of life events, Holmes and Rahe (1967) ranked in order the most stressful event (death of a spouse) to the least stressful event (minor violations of the law). These, at times, can be overpowering and stress from these events can lead to distress. If these stressors are not controlled or resolved, they have the potential to undermine the person's psychological ability to cope and could lead to despair. The literature has for a long time offered many examples of life events that cause distress and that have resulted in the person self-harming and or attempting suicide. For example, early researchers found that there was a greater than average incidence of unemployment, overcrowded living conditions, divorce and antisocial behaviour in a group of persons who were admitted to hospital after harming themselves in some way (Morgan *et al.*, 1975). Recently, it has been reported that daily stresses can trigger self-harm in young people (MHF/CF, 2006).

As noted earlier, depression can result from adverse life events, such as important circumstances that have gone wrong in the person's social environment. Very seldom are these circumstances of a medical or biological nature and frequently they lead to crisis and sometimes result in self-harm, attempted suicide or suicide. Sometimes these difficult life events are referred to as psychosocial difficulties. A psychosocial difficulty 'is any life event that could result in difficulty in coping and that could precipitate suicide-related behaviour' (McLaughlin, 1997a, p. 86). Describing all known examples of psychosocial difficulties is beyond the remit of this book. However, some of the more common have been mentioned earlier and a few more are mentioned here in brief.

Quite possibly one of the most frequent stress-inducing antecedents of suicide-related behaviour is that of interpersonal difficulties in relationships (DoH, 2001). Interpersonal difficulty is a consistent indicator of both self-harm and suicide and is therefore a major area of concern. For example, Vincent van Gogh (1853–1890) is acknowledged as a world famous painter. His paintings such *The Starry Night*, *The Sunflowers* and his haunting self-portraits have stirred the thoughts of millions of people. His brilliance as an artist is well recognized on a global scale. However, behind his expertise there is a tragic story of broken relationships, crushed emotions, sexually transmitted disease and eventually mental health problems. Vincent van Gogh was very unlucky in loving relationships. All too often it seemed that he was drawn to women who were in distress or who needed help. To some people, like his common-law wife Sien, he became a protector or others could describe him as a knight in shining armour. However, Sien had a history of prostitution and as a result of pressure from his family he had to give her up. In addition, he faced humiliation when he was rejected in other relationships. When one examines the paintings of Van Gogh, it is easy to note that a number of them reflect personal grief and misery and his famous self-portrait is very suggestive of a man in great despair. It is generally believed that his relationship difficulties contributed in some way to the development of his problems in his mental health and to his eventual suicide.

It is well known that the path of true love has never run smoothly for anyone. This saying can also be applied to difficulties in relationships in families, in heterosexual relationships and in gay and lesbian relationships (Catalan, 1983; D'Augelli and Hershberger, 1993; Morrison and L'Heureux, 2001). In addition, from a global and international perspective the empirical literature has for a very long time abounded with numerous other examples (Hawton *et al.*, 1982; Pillay, 1987; Silove, George and Bhavani-Sankaram, 1987; Platt *et al.*, 1988; Pillay and Vawda, 1989; Pan and Lieh-Mak, 1989; Jianlin, 1993; Nordentoft and Rubin, 1993; Carrigan, 1994; Hawton *et al.*, 1995; Jones, 1996; Gould *et al.*, 1996; Burgess, Hawton and Loveday, 1998; Dorer *et al.*, 1999; Hawton *et al.*, 2000; DoH, 2001).

Furthermore, a sequential pattern of interpersonal difficulty from early childhood can result in depression and lead to self-harm and suicide in later life (Silov, George and Bhavani-Sankaram, 1987; McLeod, 1991; Carrigan, 1994; Jones, 1996; Libberton, 1996). Also, the abused partner of an alcoholic may exhibit suicide-related behaviour as an escape from their plight (Pillay and Vawda, 1989). Finally, it has long been known that interpersonal relationship difficulties and particularly marriage breakdown and divorce are connected to suicide-related behaviour (DoH, 1993, 2001). Major stressors tend to come to a head around the time that a break-up of the relationship is imminent and more particularly when divorce is looming.

Other stressful life events include unemployment (Platt and Kreitman, 1990; Pritchard, 1992, 1995); sexual or gender identity (Catalan, 1983; Remafedi, Farrow and Deisher, 1991; Skegg, Nada-Raja and Dickson, 2003); and physical or sexual abuse (Riggs, Alariom and McHorneym, 1990; van Egmond *et al.*, 1993; Romans, Martin and Anderson, 1995; Davidson *et al.*, 1996; Brodsky *et al.*, 2001; Noll *et al.*, 2003; Gladstone *et al.*, 2004; Weaver *et al.*, 2004). In addition, people with eating disorders such as bulimia nervosa and anorexia nervosa are at high risk of self-harm (Paul *et al.*, 2002); in some cases anorexia can eventually result in death.

The consumption of alcohol is a sociable activity for many people. However, alcohol is a neurological depressant and when combined with psychosocial difficulties and clinical depression, there is a potential for suicide-related behaviour. It has been reported that alcohol is frequently used in combination with other drugs (Murphy, McAleer and O'Connor, 1984), thereby increasing the potential for suicidal death (Hawton, 1994a). Also, other authors confirm that substance misuse (alcohol or drugs, or both) is associated with self-harm and with suicide (De Moore and Robertson, 1996; DoH, 2001). Some people have difficulty in managing their drinking habits. For example, with the current use of closed-circuit television in many towns the media such as newspapers and television in both Great Britain and in Ireland regularly report on public demonstrations of aggression fuelled by both alcohol and other drugs in young people. Similarly, the media also show incidents where young people both openly and publicly misuse alcohol or are intoxicated in public places. In addition, one early study reported that there were 40 000 problem drinkers in Northern Ireland and of these 11 339 could be alcoholics (Blaney and MacKenzie, 1978). At that time, this equated to 1 in 25 adults in Northern Ireland. In recent times the Health Promotion Agency for Northern Ireland (HPANI) reported that some 54% of males and 41% of females in their survey reported themselves as moderate drinkers but on analysis found that they were drinking to risk or dangerous level in the week prior to the survey (HPANI, 2002).

In addition, the Health Promotion Agency for Northern Ireland (HPANI, 2003) revealed that in Northern Ireland 83% of adults aged 30–44 years drink alcohol and of this number over half the men and a third of the women were binge drinkers. Their research also found that there were many people who did not know what a binge drinking session equated to. The Health Promotion Agency define binge drinking as consuming at least 10 units of alcohol for men (approximately five drinks) and at least seven units of alcohol for women (approximately four drinks) in a single session, in other words half the recommended weekly limit. Qualitative responses to their survey found that participants interpreted binge drinking as including 'a binge is when you drink for three or four days'; 'if you take 15–20 drinks in one go'; or 'drinking to the point when you don't remember anything'.

The UK government have estimated that 15 % of people who abuse alcohol are at risk of suicide (DoH, 1993, 2001). Also, it has been suggested that having recent negative life events is a risk factor for secondary depression and suicide in male alcoholics (Roy, 1996). Therefore, people with a history of alcohol misuse are at risk of self-harm and suicide (Hawton, Fagg and McKeown, 1989; Stack and Wasserman, 1995). However, in contrast, there is another group of people who may use alcohol in their suicide-related behaviour. From an anecdotal viewpoint, I have personally worked with people who have never in their lives had a history of either using or misusing alcohol or other drugs. However, these people on the night of their suicide-related behaviour actually used either alcohol or another drug to give them 'dutch courage' in order to make the act easier. Quite possibly such anecdotal comments may be borne out with research findings in the future.

Coming to terms with one's sexual or gender identity can also precipitate self-harm and suicide in a person. This is particularly difficult for those persons who view themselves to be gay or lesbian (Catalan, 1983; Remafedi, Farrow and Deisher, 1991; Skegg, Nada-Raja and Dickson, 2003). In addition, being accepted by others, such as family and friends, is a major area of concern within this group (Rivers, 1997). Another stressful life event is physical or sexual abuse in childhood. This series of traumatic events is associated with suicide-related behaviour in adulthood (Riggs, Alariom and McHorneym, 1990; van Egmond et al., 1993; Romans, Martin and Anderson, 1995; Gladstone et al., 2004; Weaver et al., 2004).

Employment correlates positively with health and it can predict a slower decline in a person's perceived health for both males and females (Ross and Mirowsky, 1995). Suicide rates are higher among the unemployed, but the relationship between suicide and unemployment is complex (Department of Health, 1993). However, it is well known that unemployment can precipitate many psychosocial difficulties and these difficulties in turn can lead to suicide-related behaviour (Hawton, Fagg and Simkin, 1988; Platt and Kreitman, 1990; Pritchard, 1992, 1995; Carrigan, 1994; Western Investment for Health, 2006). While Pritchard (1992) found that increases in the male suicide rate were statistically associated with unemployment, Owen and Watson (1995) suggest that the link between unemployment and poor mental health is not clear. For example, is unemployment the cause of poor mental health or a result of poor mental health? It is well recognized that unemployment will more than likely restrict a person's spending power. The person will probably have less money to live on and to live in the style to which they had become accustomed. Shortage of finance can curtail a person's social interactions and it may result in their withdrawal from family and friends. A downward spiral may ensue and if the person does not regain new employment within a year it may impact on their mental health. This downward spiral can be accelerated if the person's family is dependent on their income. For instance, how can a family go out together if they cannot afford it? How can they afford to pay the mortgage, put food on the table, entertain friends, go on holidays, hold birthday parties, buy presents, celebrate Christmas or other similar festive occasions? The inability to afford such activities may create stress on the person to provide for their family. It may also create interpersonal relationship difficulties within the family. Such stress can become compounded by other negative emotional responses such as arguments among family members, feelings of shame or guilt within the family. If not resolved these difficulties may become worse and have the potential to lead to crisis. For instance, in a recent study it was reported that one in five unemployed men seriously thought about suicide (WIH, 2006). Thus, there may be an indirect relationship between unemployment and suicide-related behaviour. In contrast, other authors have reported that where unemployment is high in a population, then unemployment status is less deviant (Platt and Kreitman, 1990) and self-harm or suicide may not be associated with it. However, in populations where unemployment is rare then one of the most important issues is the person's and particularly the family's ability to cope and respond to unemployment. If unemployment adversely affects the family and they are unable to cope, then this may cause distress in the main breadwinner. If financial resources diminish and the prospects of re-employment fade, then interpersonal difficulties and disharmony within the family unit may develop. In turn, hopelessness or despair about the future is very likely and the potential for crisis is very real.

Furthermore, the exploration of the effects of 'daily hassles' on a person's mental and physical health has added to the stressful life events perspective. Daily hassles are those 'irritating, frustrating, or distressing incidents that occur in our everyday transactions with the environment' (Lazarus, 1981, p. 58). This statement can also apply to a person's interactions with other people such as work colleagues. Although a small sample was used (n = 100) and the results could not be generalized, Lazarus (1981) found that stressful life events did have some long-term effects, but in the short term, hassles seem to have a much stronger impact on mental and physical health. For example, how would you feel if a colleague took time off work and left this work for you to do? Another example could be where colleagues do not do their job correctly and leave another colleague to tidy up their mess. Similarly, having an argument with a work colleague, friend or family member can easily become a hassle. Such hassles can eventually become overpowering and may impact on a person's mental health more so than other, what may be termed, major life events. In themselves daily hassles may not result in suicide-related behaviour but when combined with other negative events in a person's life, they may wear the person's mental resilience down and crisis may occur. For example, if a person is having difficulties in their relationships at home and then is subjected to 'daily hassles' at work, this could create negative thoughts about the future. Indeed, when the future looks bleak or seems hopeless then suicide-related behaviour may become an option.

The above are only a few examples of life events that may precede either self-harm or suicide. Overall, it seems that any adverse major life event can trigger either self-harm or suicide. If a person cannot cope with difficult life events then self-harm or suicide may become an option. For example, Linehan *et al.* (1987) assert that where problem-solving deficits occur, combined with lack of assertiveness, then self-harming behaviour is high. This does not imply that people avoid problem solving; rather they are affected by the outcomes of their problem-solving efforts (Thoits, 1994). Failed problem-solving attempts can intensify a person's distress and could induce negative thoughts affecting self-esteem and the person's control of their psychosocial difficulties (Lazarus, 1993). Indeed, McLaughlin, Miller and Warwick (1996) reported that self-harm was likely when a person has exhausted their problem-solving abilities.

While various adverse life events may thus lead to self-harm and to suicide, it has been suggested that hopelessness about the future is the link between adverse life events and the resultant behaviour. For example, hopelessness in people correlates highly with self-harm (McLaughlin, Miller and Warwick, 1996) and with the intention to kill themselves (Beck, Kovacs and Weissman, 1975; Beck *et al.*, 1985; McLaughlin, Miller and Warwick, 1996; Bolland, 2003). Thus, it seems that suicide-related behaviour is very likely when a person is pessimistic about their future.

Also, a number of authors suggest that self-harm is a form of communication to others that a person cannot cope with a life event and is facing an intolerable amount of psychache (McLaughlin, Miller and Warwick, 1996; Dorer *et al.*, 1999). For many, self-harm is an escape from this psychache, or a way of drawing attention to events causing the psychache (Dorer *et al.*, 1999). In many of these cases self-harm, rather than suicide, is the response. However where the stressor is of perceived greater difficulty, combined with hopelessness about the future, or where previous self-harming behaviour provoked an unsympathetic response, then suicide or attempted suicide may occur.

The empirical evidence shows that negative life events are stressors and are prime risk factors for and precipitate psychache and suicide-related behaviour. It is important to note that, unlike Freud's or Erikson's theories, most of the above examples reflect recent crises, rather than deep-rooted emotional despair emanating from childhood experiences. The stressful life-events perspective, while providing an insight into the downward spiral towards suicide-related behaviour, can also lend itself very much towards the required therapeutic approach needed to help a person through their crisis.

(g) The social integration perspective

All of the previous perspectives are psychological. However, Durkheim (1897/1951) explains suicide from a sociological perspective. Durkheim's study is a classic and it was a first major attempt to associate the occurrence of suicide with events that were happening in the wider society. Even though Durkheim's study has been criticized by a number of authors, it still remains influential to this day. It would be difficult for any author to consider suicide and its related behaviour without first visiting some of the influential points that Durkheim made in his study. A fundamental belief in Durkheim's study is that major changes in social circumstances are a main precipitating factor in suicide. For instance, two of Durkheim's classifications of suicide are: (1) anomic suicide where a person feels isolated as a result of social fragmentation or sudden change in their status in society; and (2) egoistic suicide where a person fails to integrate with society.

Anomic suicide: The term anomie literally means 'without norms'. Frequently, anomie is associated with social fragmentation or social deregulation. For instance, some would consider high divorce rates in a country as a sign of social fragmentation. It would follow that where a suicide occurs as a result of divorce or separation then it could be classified as an 'anomic suicide'. In recent times, the Institute for Public Policy Research (IPPR, 2006) have expressed concern at the way society, particularly in the United Kingdom, is raising its children. They (IPPR, 2006) suggest that the role of government in supporting children is out of date and that changes to the family structure have undermined the ability of the family to socialize their children effectively. An underpinning thought in this research is the concern that children may have greater difficulty in problem solving during their adult years. Given that difficulty in problem solving is linked to suicide-related behaviour, there is a possibility that suicide-related behaviour might be linked to child-rearing practices in society.

However, anomic suicide can also occur when there is a sudden or unexpected change in the person's life. For example, the person may be overwhelmed and unable to cope with sudden difficulties that life brings. For instance, they may feel in danger, threatened, or that they no longer serve a useful purpose in society. The extended family living together is currently a rare event. Many children now move away from home leaving parents on their own. In addition, people die or move away and the society that person grew up in changes. New people come along and they bring new attitudes and possibly even fear. This can be difficult for some people to accept. Also, more often than not, a person's difficulties will involve sudden loss. This loss will bring about changes in the person's relationship with society. For instance, a person may become bankrupt and this could impact very heavily on the mental health and physical well-being of them and their immediate family. Young people may be able to build their lives again after bank-ruptcy but some middle- or older-aged people may find it difficult in coping with bankruptcy. During the great depression in the USA (1929) many people killed themselves after they lost their personal wealth. Also, a number of those who survived the concentration camps and the holocaust during World War II eventu-ally killed themselves. Strangely enough, anomic suicide can also apply to people who come into unexpected wealth.

Egoistic suicide: In egoistic suicide some people fail to develop or keep close relationships in society. In the present day many people, especially young people, are very mobile. Also, the extended family and the sense of belonging to a community rarely exist now. A classic example is a person who leaves home and travels to a new country or larger city. Quite possibly the person may fail to maintain contacts with family and with friends at home and may eventually lose all contact. This in turn would result in the loss of social support for the person, isolation and possible alienation from other people. For instance, in Case vignette 4 Stephen's suicide-related behaviour resulted from a combination of him finding that his partner was unfaithful and that he had no real friends or any other support network where he was living. In addition, Hawton (1993) sug-gested that the high rise in suicide in young males might have resulted from young men becoming less integrated with society and supported by those around them with the reverse in women. In Durkheim's (1897/1951) theory, it is sug-gested that the more integrated a society is and the more integrated a person is into a society, the lower the incidence of suicide in that society. In recent times it has been reported that many young people who self-harm feel socially isolated (MHF/CF, 2006).

Altruistic suicide: This is where the person kills him or herself as an act for a greater good. Within their own societies this type of suicide may be viewed favourably. An example of altruistic suicide would be the hunger strikers who died during the 'Troubles' in Northern Ireland. Also, and as mentioned earlier the Japanese kamikaze pilots during World War II and the 'suicide bombers' in the conflicts in Iraq and in Afghanistan.

Much of social integration theory revolves around the social support net-works of a person. Speck (1967) suggested that social support networks include family, relatives, friends and fellow workers with whom a person interacts. Turner and Marino (1994) found that the epidemiology of perceived social support cor-responded closely with the epidemiology of distress and that women had a high level of perceived social support. Rigby (2000) suggests that poor social support contributes towards adolescents' poor mental health. In addition, Hawton (1994b) suggests that the high levels of support available to young women may protect them from suicide, but that young men who lack social support may be prone to suicide.

De Wilde *et al.* (1994) found that a 'high-risk' group of adolescent suicide attempters were different from a psychologically 'normal' group because they reported less support from siblings and relations outside the family. These authors also report that their high-risk group relied on social networks outside the family. Similarly, Conrad (1992) and Boldero and Fallon (1995) also reported that adolescents relied on friends when facing interpersonal difficulties. In brief, all persons are exposed to stressful life events and social networks provide support for them, promote mental health, and buffer distress (Lazarus, 1981; Greenblath, *et al.*, 1982; Cohen and Wills, 1985; Conrad, 1991; Heikkinen *et al.*, 1993; Thoits, 1994). In effect, it seems that social support here is a mechanism for preventing the development of despair and therefore has the potential to prevent suicide-related behaviour. However, in contrast, the absence of a social network or a perceived absence of a social network in a person's life could compound psychosocial difficulties, increase feelings of isolation and eventually result in self-harm or in suicide.

(h) The mental ill-health perspective

It is well recognized that people who have a history of mental ill-health are disproportionately at higher risk of suicide-related behaviour than those in other groups. In addition, mental ill-health is predicated to become the greatest burden of disease in the developed world for the next two decades (WHO, 2001, 2002a). Also, the World Health Organization (WHO, 2001) suggested that mental ill-health is one of the leading causes of disability worldwide and amounts to a huge cost in terms of human unhappiness, disability and economic loss. Of all the serious forms of mental ill-health, depression and schizophrenia are the most prominent at risk of suicide (King, 1994; Royal College of Psychiatrists, 1996; Rihmer, 1996; DoH, 2001). Other groups at risk are people diagnosed as neurotic, abusing alcohol or other drugs, and particularly people diagnosed as having a personality disorder (Ahrens and Haug, 1996). A brief review of the literature pertaining to depression and schizophrenia will highlight the importance of each.

Depression as a risk factor

Depression is the commonest of all the psychiatric disorders (Seligman, 1975; Andrew *et al.*,1993). It is sub-classified in a number of ways and distinctions have to be made between endogenous or clinical depression and exogenous or reactive depression (Duffield, 1992). In brief, endogenous depression is likely to originate from a biological perspective in which a neurochemical dysfunction in one of the neurotransmitters such as serotonin, acetylcholine, norepinephrine, dopamine and gamma-aminobutyric acid (GABA) is implicated. Much of the discussion surrounding these neurotransmitters can be found under the biological perspective in this chapter. In contrast, exogenous depression originates from psychosocial stressors such as conflict with a partner or loss of a job. The theoretical perspectives underpinning these psychosocial difficulties or stressors have also been discussed previously in this chapter. Although exogenous depression seems to be less severe than endogenous depression, the experience of exogenous depression can be very disturbing and, at the extreme, it can be a precipitant of suicide-related behaviour (Pritchard, 1995).

Depression has been estimated as accounting for 75% of all psychiatric admissions (Boyd and Weissman, 1982) and the rate of depression among women in western industrialized nations was estimated as being almost twice the rate among men (Brown and Harris, 1978). Also, the risk of suicide is high in endogenous depression (King, 1994; Malone *et al.*, 1995; RCP, 1996; Foster, Gillespie and McClelland, 1997; DoH, 2001). According to the Department of Health (2001) some 45% of their sample were diagnosed as suffering from bipolar affective disorder at the time of their suicide. The precipitating factors of depression are many and no single factor can explain the onset of depression; rather depression can result from an interaction between a variety of factors that include biological, environmental, psychosocial and family history. These factors are similar to many of those that precipitate suicide-related behaviour.

Most people experience episodes of low mood, which are transient, but can disturb many aspects of daily functioning. However, clinical depression endures for a longer time-span. In clinical depression, people are usually troubled with guilt and anxiety is increased, they become more irritable than usual, and find it difficult to enjoy normal daily activities. In addition, a clinically depressed person frequently lacks motivation, has low energy and feels that everything is an effort. Usually a depressed person will withdraw from social contact and spend much time alone being preoccupied with negative thoughts. They neglect their social networks and harmony within the family is affected (Badger, 1996). Bodily functions, sleep, appetite and sexual desire are usually disturbed as a result of morbid thoughts. Barraclough and Pallis (1975) have reported that compared with a control group, depressed people who killed themselves had more persistent insomnia, were more agitated, manifested more self-neglect, had more impairment of memory and had made previous suicide attempts. Characteristically, they were older, male, single or separated/divorced and more socially isolated.

While depression has poor links with self-harm (McLaughlin, Miller and Warwick, 1996; NICE, 2004a), it is well linked to attempted suicide (Silver *et al.*, 1971). However, Wilkinson (1989) reports that only 15% of depressed persons eventually kill themselves by suicide. Thus, most depressed persons, even if they at some times have suicide-related ideation, do not progress to suicide. The link between depression and suicide is thus not clear-cut. In the past a number of famous people, such as the painter Vincent Van Gogh and the comedian Peter Sellers, have had histories of severe depression. Also, in recent times, the mass media regularly reports on the personal lives of celebrities. Quite a number of celebrities such as Robbie Williams (singer), Linda Hamilton (actress), Jim Carrey (actor), Ben Stiller (actor), and Winona Ryder (actress) have shared their experiences of depression with the public in the media. However, in some cases prolonged depression can result in hopelessness about the future (Beck *et al.*, 1974; MacLeod, Rose and Williams, 1993), which in turn is linked to increased risk of suicide (Fremouw, Callahan and Kashden, 1993; Hawton, 1994b), and self-harm or suicide (Beck *et al.*, 1993; Bolland, 2003). Therefore, when depression is accompanied by hopelessness or pessimism about the future, then self-harm or suicide is very likely. In addition, a previous history of self-harm (Kelleher *et al.*, 2000) or attempted suicide (Nordstrom *et al.*, 1995; Brádvik, 2003) in depressed persons is a strong indicator of future suicide.

The person experiencing severe depression is in an awful mental place. Frequently the feelings that are experienced in depression are called 'The Blues'. This is probably some form of tribute towards the colours that Vincent Van Goth used in paintings when he was depressed. However, the reality is that the feelings experienced in severe depression are much worse than 'The Blues'. For example, Redfield-Jamison (1995) describes it as awful beyond words in which the person is unable to enjoy life, lacks confidence and self-respect, is unable to think normally and has both day and night terrors. These emotions can become so intense that the person finds the emotional pain (psychache) of it too much to bear. In an effort to escape this psychache, or in trying to end it, the person may consider suicide-related behaviour.

Schizophrenia as a risk factor

Schizophrenics are vulnerable to depression (Gillman and Wilson, 1996; Harkavy-Friedman *et al.*, 2004) and a substantial number attempt suicide at some stage in their illness (Roy, Mazonson and Pickar, 1984; McGlashan, 1984; Chatterton, 1995). Some researchers have reported that even when depression, hopelessness, substance abuse and social problem solving were controlled for, there was a significant link between psychotic disorder and suicide-related ideation (Warman *et al.*, 2004). Also, almost 10 % of chronic schizophrenics end their lives by suicide (Roy, Mazonson and Pickar, 1984). Additionally, the Royal College of Psychiatrists (1996) reported that just over 25% of the people who killed themselves by suicide were diagnosed as experiencing schizophrenia. More recently, a five-year follow up of this study revealed that approximately 20% of their sample who died by suicide were diagnosed as schizophrenics (DoH, 2001). It has also been reported that a number of people who have had a diagnosis of schizophrenia die by suicide within a short period of being discharged (DoH, 2001; Pirkola, Sohlman and

Wahlbeck, 2005). Most of the persons who died by suicide had recorded some improvement in their mental well-being prior to discharge. Also, it has been reported that patients with schizophrenia were found to attempt suicide more early in their lives than patients with mood disorders (Ran *et al.*, 2004). Furthermore, in a systematic review of the literature carried out by Haw *et al.* (2005) they report that people diagnosed with schizophrenia are also prone to acts of self-harm.

Suicide in schizophrenics occurs mainly during non-psychotic phases in their illness. For instance some reports make the point that the person had shown improvement in their mental health status prior to their discharge (DoH, 2001; Pirkola, Sohlman and Wahlbeck, 2005). Frequently the person would have attained a high level of education and were very much aware of the effects of schizophrenia and its consequences in later life. However, some authors have reported that contrary to expectations, general awareness of the mental disorder did not predict suicide (Amador *et al.*, 1996). Suicide is less likely to occur during acute florid psychosis (Drake and Cotton, 1986) and the presence of command hallucinations was not associated with greater suicidal risk (Wilkinson and Bacon, 1984). However, depression, feelings of inadequacy, hopelessness and suicide-related ideation in schizophrenics can indicate future self-harm and suicide (Westermeyer and Harrow, 1989; Harkavy-Friedman *et al.*, 2004). While this may be so, both Yarden (1974) and King (1994) agree that few schizophrenics give warnings of suicidal intent and that 'these suicides are seldom preceded by the signals given by persons in other diagnostic groups' (King, 1994, p. 661). Nonetheless, mental health practitioners must recognize and be aware that persons experiencing schizophrenia do face additional emotional and psychological difficulties in their lives. These difficulties can and do lead the person experiencing schizophrenia to consider suicide-related behaviour as a method of coping or a permanent resolution to their difficulties (Harkavy-Friedman *et al.*, 2004; Pirkola, Sohlman and Wahlbeck, 2005; Haw *et al.*, 2005).

Personality disorder as a risk factor

Of all the diagnoses used in psychiatry, personality disorder is one of the most disputed (Pembroke, 1998a, 1998b). In general, whenever personality traits are rigid, impair judgement or functioning and lead to distress, then a diagnosis of personality disorder is likely. Included within the diagnosis of personality disorder is psychopathic disorder. Other personality disorders are outlined by Tyrer (2000) and include: antisocial, borderline, narcissistic and dependent. In fact clinical definitions can range from the most timid to the most violent in society. The Mental Health Act (England and Wales) in 1983 addresses psychopathic disorder in Sections 3, 37 and 47. Also, the term psychopathic disorder, according to the

Department of Health and the Home Office (DoH, 1994) describes a number of 'personality disorders'. However, it is worthwhile noting that there is no legal classification of psychopathic disorder or of personality disorder in either the Mental Health (Scotland) Act (1984) or in the Mental Health (Northern Ireland) Order (1986). Because of this, measuring the prevalence of personality disorders is very difficult. However, according to the National Institute for Mental Health in England (NIMHE, 2003) between 36% and 67% of inpatients were diagnosed as having a personality disorder.

According to Castillo, Allen and Coxhead (2001) the diagnosis of personality disorder has a stigmatizing effect on the person. For example, any person using a library or the Internet can access the definitions in the ICD-10 (WHO, 1992) or in the DSM-IV (American Psychiatric Association, 2000). They will find that personality disorders include terms such as long-lasting, rigid or inflexible personality traits. These can suggest no help, no cure and no hope for the future. In addition, Castillo, Allen and Coxhead (2001) report that 72% of their sample (n = 50) had experienced bad treatment as a result of their diagnosis. This is coupled with the knowledge that 80% of the same sample had experienced abuse in childhood. However, while abuse in childhood may be associated with many people who self-harm, Pembroke (1998a, 1998b) urges caution in trying to fix a 'one cause to fit all'. Nonetheless, for many of those in Castillo et al.'s (2001) sample, especially those who were abused as children, behaviours such as self-harm, substance and medicine misuse were employed as coping mechanisms and as a means of gaining some control over their lives. Again it seems that self-harm is being used as a form of communicating the despair that the person is experiencing. While the link between self-harm and people who are classified as having a personality disorder is acknowledged in this book, this does not mean that the author agrees with or accepts the concept of personality disorder as a psychiatric diagnosis.

Crisis

The term crisis comes from the Greek word *krisis*, which means decision. The Concise Oxford English Dictionary (Sykes, 1987) defines it as a 'time of danger'. In addition, there is a word of warning as the two Chinese symbols that represent crisis mean 'danger' and 'opportunity' respectively. There is very little difference between a suicidal crisis and a crisis that does not include suicide-related behaviour. The only difference is that in one case the person has decided that suicide-related behaviour is a potential solution to their crisis. Therefore, when a crisis is reached, the person will decide on a course of action. While a crisis can occur at any time in a person's life, it is more likely to occur at a point when it seems to the person that they need to take some action. Crisis is the point where a person is liable to break down and become disorganized (Caplan, 1964). At this point the person's usual coping strategies have been overwhelmed, have become exhausted or have failed. Frequently, crisis is the point where a person's behaviour changes. Considering all that a person has gone through before they reached a crisis point (see Figure 5.1), how do professional health carers think a person would feel after making previous failed attempts to resolve the stressor in their life? Many practitioners will find this question very difficult to answer, because emotions are very personal to each person who is experiencing a crisis. Therefore, dealing with stressors will be very individual and very personal to each person. It is worth remembering that Lazarus (1993) makes the point that failing to resolve stressors will increase the person's distress.

A crisis situation in anyone's life can result in any number of behavioural or psychological responses. These responses can have either positive or negative effects on the person. For example, some responses would include seeking professional help and developing problem-solving strategies. It will be very obvious to practitioners that the person should have employed this type of response as early as possible and especially before their difficulty became a crisis. Unfortunately, this obviousness is not always apparent in the person who is now experiencing crisis. It has previously been reported that some people, especially adolescents, have difficulty in seeking professional help (Woods, 1990; Boldero and Fallon, 1995) and in engaging them in therapy (Dorer et al., 1999). Also, scrutiny of the government annual numbers of recorded suicides in both Great Britain and in the island of Ireland show that young males in the 15–25-year-old age group are four times more likely to kill themselves by suicide than females. The assumption here is that males generally have difficulty in talking about their psychological difficulties. Therefore, a good number of males may have no contact with practitioners, whether statutary or voluntary, until they have reached crisis point. However, even in a crisis situation, some people will still find it difficult to share their feelings with another human being. Even so, seeking professional help can be the first step in resolving or at least reducing the effects of the stressor. If the outcome of a person's response to the crisis is positive, then the person will learn a more positive way to help himself in the future.

In contrast, the response by some people to crisis could include misusing alcohol or drugs, venting one's feelings in a violent way on family members or friends, or harming themselves in some way. While catharsis, the expression of emotions, may seem to be a good form of therapy, taking out one's negative emotions in a violent way on the self, the family or on friends will most certainly not develop harmonious relationships within the family or peers. Similarly, the misuse of alcohol or drugs in attempting to support the person in times of stress may result in additional difficulties and strained interpersonal relationships. At a time of crisis, other responses could include suicide-related behaviour such as self-harm and suicide. Whether or not we as practitioners agree, all of these responses can bring about a temporary or, in the case of suicide, permanent reprieve from the stressor. However, in self-harm the reprieve is usually brief and it is not a permanent solution. Negative responses may initially seem positive to the person because they bring about such a temporary relief from the stressor. It has been reported that in some cases adolescents have evaluated that their self-harming behaviour (overdosing) helped them (Hawton *et al.*, 1982; Burgess, Hawton and Loveday, 1998; Dorer *et al.*, 1999). However, Burgess, Hawton and Loveday (1998) warn that in their sample, all had taken an overdose for the first time and that reactions towards the person and their behaviour may be less positive if they repeated the behaviour in the future. Thus, these types of responses to crisis can eventually impact negatively on the person and on other people who are significant in the person's life. Previous supportive relationships may be damaged as a direct result of a person's negative or maladaptive responses to a stressor. Where relationships have been negatively affected and particularly during a time of crisis, the person may feel very much alone and overwhelmed by the effects of the stressor. At such times a person in crisis may feel that they have no one else to turn to for help and suicide-related behaviour could very well become an option.

From a psychological point of view, human beings evaluate their progress in life and the outcomes of various life events. When the effects of a stressor have been resolved or at least reduced, the person will more than likely evaluate their responses in a positive way and possibly use what they have learned in future similar situations. However, how would a person, who is in crisis, evaluate their behavioural response that has not resolved nor reduced the effects of the stressor? Such an evaluation would compound a crisis. We must remember that people are affected by the outcomes of their problem-solving efforts (Thoits, 1994). For example, a person's evaluation of him or herself, particularly if it is a negative valuation, may complicate and add to any previous feelings of depression, low self-esteem, worthlessness, helplessness and quite possibly hopelessness or despair. At this point, a decision has to be made about the way forward; the person may, if they have not done so before, decide to talk to others such as family, friends and professional health carers. Also, it is possible that they may decide on some other behavioural response such as self-harm or suicide.

Summary of stressors leading to suicide-related behaviour

In summary, stressors that lead to distress, crisis and suicide-related behaviour can emanate from many different sources. For instance, in much the way that the city of Rome can be viewed differently from each of its hills, each of the preceding perspectives offer differing viewpoints as to how a person may arrive at the point of crisis. The sources of stressors are many and they can arise from within the person as in the biological perspective or from an external source as in many of the other perspectives. Each perspective has in common the notion of conflict or crisis arising at some point in the person's life. For example, biological dysfunction, early childhood experiences, or current psychosocial difficulties can lead to distress and these in turn can lead to negative thoughts about the self and the future. As indicated in Figure 5.1, such thoughts, if uncontrolled and if the difficulties are not resolved, can lead the person to despair about the future. When stressors are unresolved then the person will more than likely experience psychache and crisis may develop. When a person reaches a crisis point, they will make a decision and a behavioural response will occur. For instance, the behavioural response could be any behaviour, no matter how radical or unusual, that will deal with or that avoids the stressor. Unfortunately in many cases the behavioural response is some form of suicide-related behaviour. In brief, the thought that is advocated in this book is that suicide-related behaviour is a person's way of communicating their psychache or deep emotional distress.

All of the perspectives mentioned previously suggest ways that distress can arise in the person and can then lead to feelings of despair. Whether or not the person effectively deals with the actual stressor is very much dependent on a number of things. Some of these are: (1) how important the stressor is to the person; (2) the person's problem-solving abilities and (3) the social support network that the person has. If unresolved, stressors can lead to despair and then develop into a crisis and the potential for self-harm and suicide can become a reality. However, just as each perspective offers rationale for the development of stressors and the beginning of the descent into crisis, all of the perspectives offer rationale for helping the person at least to cope and possibly resolve their crisis. Later in this book we will revisit some of the issues in these perspectives in order to consider how practitioners can respond to a person who is considering suicide-related behaviour.

Responding to crisis

6

In Chapter 6 the following issues are explored:

1. A person's response to crisis
2. The biological response to stressors
3. Coping abilities as buffers against stressors
4. Cognitive and emotional responses as buffers against stressors
5. Social support as a buffer against stressors
6. Positive attitude as a buffer against stressors
7. Individual differences as buffers against stressors
8. The person's behavioural response to crisis
9. Help-seeking behaviour – contact with the caring services
10. Stressor resolved
11. Stressor unresolved – crisis

A person's response to crisis

Every event or incident that causes stress in a person will produce a response or a series of responses within the person. For instance, some people will reach a certain point of tolerance where they will respond in a very forthright manner that will resolve or develop some coping mechanism that deals with whatever is causing them distress or despair. In all cases, everyone who has ever felt distress in their lives will have felt the body's physiological response to distress. This physiological response to stress creates feelings of anxiety in a person and on occasion these become too much for the person. However, it is well known that the physiological effects may be somewhat relieved by a medical response. For example, in order to reduce the physical feelings of stress and anxiety, the GP may prescribe a short course of anxiolytic medication. However, while such medication may reduce the physiological response to a stressor, there is not a pill for every ill. In other words, stressors cannot be resolved by purely biological or medical responses. Therefore, along with the physiological response, the person will call upon his or her psychological support defences or social network system in order to resolve or at least buffer the effect of the stressor. Some of these buffers include the person's coping abilities, cognitive and emotional responses, social support networks, positive attitude and other individual differences (Cohen and Wills, 1985; Cohen and Herbert, 1996).

The effect that psychological buffers have in moderating the potential harmful effects of stressors is important. For example, the physiological response will physically prepare the person for the stressor but will not necessarily on its own produce an actual solution. The unfortunate side of this is that the body could eventually use up all its physical resources without resolving the stressor. This could have a devastating effect on the person. However, the psychological response, with support from the physiological response can produce potential and permanent solutions. Nonetheless, if the psychological buffers can moderate, minimize, or deal effectively with the stressor then the person's coping mechanisms are sound. In this case the ill effects on the person, both physical and psychological, will be avoided and feelings of despair will be prevented.

The biological response to stressors

It has long been known that the body can respond in a biological manner to threat or potential threat from a physical or psychological stressor. This response is a mobilization of the body's physiological defence systems. During this response the body tends to respond in what is termed a 'fight or flight response' (Cannon, 1929). In this response the hypothalamus stimulates the adrenal medulla, through the sympathetic nervous system, to secrete epinephrine (adrenaline) and norepinephrine (noradrenaline). The effect of these hormones is an increased cardiovascular response, increased respiration, increased blood flow to the muscles and increased mental activity. At the same time the hypothalamus stimulates the pituitary gland to release corticotrophin, which in turn stimulates the adrenal cortex to secrete corticosteroids. The effect of the corticosteroids on the body is to increase protein and fat metabolism, increase access to stored energy and to decrease the body's normal inflammatory response. Normally the mobilization of the body's natural defence forces is not in any way harmful as the parasympathetic nervous system calms the arousal associated with the sympathetic system. However, as shown in Figure 5.1, if this physiological response and increased state of awareness is prolonged, then the effects on the person could lead to both physical and psychological exhaustion. For example, according to Selye (1956) the body can undergo three stages of physiological reactions in response to stress. Selye (1956) called these reactions the General Adaptation Syndrome (GAS).

The first stage of the General Adaptation Syndrome is the 'fight or flight response' (Cannon, 1929) or as (Selye, 1956) called it the 'alarm reaction'. As outlined above the body prepares to meet the threat or demand by mobilizing its defences through the sympathetic nervous system. In addition, the body will also call upon psychological support defences to solve or cushion the effects of the stressor prior to the full advent of the physiological response. In the alarm reaction stage, if the stressor has been successfully dealt with, the normal physiological response is that the parasympathetic nervous system will relax and calm the physiological reactions.

However, if the effects of the stressor persist, the body's response enters a second stage called 'resistance'. In this stage the physiological responses that were mobilized in the alarm reaction stage are enhanced, strengthened, and maintained. The full advent of the physiological response will continue until the effects of the stressor are minimized or overcome. Alternatively, the physiological response, in the absence of a solution to the effects of the stressor, will increase and the person's body will enter the third and final stage called 'exhaustion'. In this stage the person's physiological and psychological defences are scarce or depleted and (s)he may show signs of physical illness, physical deterioration and mental exhaustion. At this stage the person may seek, temporary or permanent, relief from their emotional turmoil, crisis may occur and suicide-related behaviour may be the response.

Coping abilities as buffers against stressors

The person's psychological ability to buffer negative effects depends very much on the exact demands of the stressor. Active coping is where the person is able to reduce their exposure to the stressor by avoiding it or escaping from it (Obrist, 1981). Also, a person's ability to cope could include dealing effectively with or overcoming the stressor. This type of coping is similar to problem-focused coping, which also includes trying to control the stressor. For example, impending exams can create anxiety in students. However, is studying for an exam an example of active or problem-focused coping? Similarly, when a person has an important meeting that could influence his or her future prospects, they may role-play the event in preparation. More often than not the astute person will practise their interview skills before attending an interview. In contrast, passive coping is where the person is unable to respond either physically or psychologically to a stressor and (s)he may simply tolerate the stressor and its effects on them. This type of response could eventually create a drain on the person's physical and psychological resources and coupled with other stressors could lead to very negative thoughts about the self. Another form of coping that would be classified as response-focused coping is where a person is made aware that an event is coming up and they perceive it as potentially stressful. The person could respond and try to reduce the anticipatory anxiety of a stressor by exercising or other physical activity. For instance, they may take part in a physically challenging activity that diverts their attention away from the negative effects of the stressors. Others may take part in some form of relaxation therapy that helps them to deal with the physical effects of the stressor.

Overall, the person's coping abilities are very important in resolving, moderating, or reducing the effects of stressors on the person. As De La Fuente (1990) reported, when people cope successfully, they can resume functioning at their pre-stressor level and in some cases they learn from their experience and grow from it. This is also evidenced in Mark's brief case history (Case vignette 22), as outlined earlier in this book, where Mark learned and grew from his experience.

Cognitive and emotional responses as buffers against stressors

Cognitive and emotional factors also play an important part in resolving, moderating or reducing the strength of a stressor. For example, cognitive appraisal (Lazarus and Folkman, 1984) is very much to the fore here. This is where the person is aware that an event, either happy (wedding) or sad (divorce), is planned. The person is made aware of the event in adequate time and has time to prepare for it. The person can appraise all aspects of the event, negative and positive, and thus reduce potential adverse psychological or physical effects. Also, the person can employ role-playing techniques as a method to deal with potential stressors. This allows the person time to think about the best way of dealing with potential stressors and possibly take preventative action or at least reduce the potential effects. However, a worst-case scenario is where an unexpected or unpredictable event occurs and the person has not had the chance to prepare for it. For example, the sudden death of a loved one or the sudden ending of a relationship can bring about severe emotional responses in a person.

Also, from a psychological point of view, the person's perceived control (Ajzen, 1985, 1988; Ajzen and Timko, 1986; Kanner and Feldman, 1991) over an event is a very important factor that can help a person deal with stressors. Being in control of an event and providing that the person has all the necessary requirements can certainly help to minimize the potential effects of adverse stressors. It is sometimes said that a potentially negative event that is controllable is less stressful than a potentially negative event that is not controllable. In addition, the power of hindsight is a powerful thing and in many cases when reviewing results people can view an uncontrollable event as being somehow controllable. For example, many people will recall times when they thought, 'If only I did that differently.' These types of thoughts can in themselves be quite stress-provoking and can lead a person to make negative assumptions about their own problem-solving abilities in times of crisis.

In a similar way, emotional responses can buffer the effects of stressors. For example, in Lazarus (1981) there is a warning that too many daily 'hassles' can become stressful and overwhelm the person. Such stressful events may occur in the home or in the workplace in the form of an argument with a partner or a work colleague. For some people, the chosen method in dealing with such an incident is to deal effectively with their own feelings. Say for example that the person feels angry, not about what was said but that the argument even started. Then the emotion-focused coping may be to deal with their feelings of anger. When the person has reduced their anger, their body should return to a state of calm again.

Social support as a buffer against stressors

A person's social support or social network can also influence the effects of stressors on the person. Durkheim (1897/1951) believed that deterioration in social circumstances was a major factor that precipitated suicide. Also, almost 100 years later, Hawton (1993) responding to a noticeable increase in the suicides of young males suggested that it may have resulted from young men becoming less integrated with society and less supported by those around them. Hawton (1993) also suggested that the lower rates of suicide in women were because women were more integrated into society.

It seems that having family, friends and significant others to socialize with, talk to or call upon in times of difficulty is a buffer against the effects of stressors in a person's life (Cohen and Wills, 1985). However, Kulik and Mahler (1993) suggest that not any old friend, spouse or partner will provide a buffer against the effects of stressors. They suggest that the personality of the support provider (friend, spouse, partner, or practitioner) will determine whether or not the person will perceive the social support as a buffer against a stressor or experience it as another source of stress. In addition, there are implications here for how the person perceives the help offered by practitioners. There is a good possibility that some practitioners are a buffer against stressors and others may not be. Nonetheless, the suggestion here is that a positive social support system and a more integrated society could buffer against the effects of stressors in the person.

Positive attitude as a buffer against stressors

According to Jahoda (1958) there are six criteria for positive mental health. Among these is the person's positive attitude towards him or herself. Having a positive attitude towards oneself involves several issues. The person must accept who they are by having a sense of their own identity. Part of this can be achieved by being successful or by belonging to a cohesive group of companions who allow each member to put forth their points of view or contribute towards the success of the group. For example, people have different roles in groups. Each role brings certain responsibilities and the success of the group depends on each member's contribution. In this way, when the group is successful in its endeavours, belonging to such a group can create a positive attitude in a person's life.

However, a positive attitude towards the self must also be coupled with realistic aspirations and expectations. The success of an event through one's efforts is a strong motivator for future activities. A powerful sense of self-efficacy comes from self-achievement, 'nothing succeeds like success' (Bandura, 1984). Being successful can develop a person's psychological well-being and also a positive attitude towards the self. It would therefore be important that in a person's self evaluation they are able to recognize the part they played in their own success. However, how success is achieved is important to the person and Murray (1947, p. 138) warns that 'when we fail in that (development) all other success is empty: for we take our pleasure without joy, and the ache of boredom warns of a rusting faculty'. Thus, it seems that a person's own evaluation of their success is crucial in how they feel about themselves.

In contrast, a person may have unrealistic aspirations and expectations. If according to Bandura (1984) that self-achievement is a powerful personal motivator, then surely failure in a number of events would decrease the person's motivation to try again. There is nothing wrong with having high aspirations or expectations about the future. It is what a person does to achieve those aspirations or expectations that matters. Failure at times can also motivate for the future, providing that the person learns and adapts from their failure. However, where repetitive failures occur, then low self-esteem and a negative attitude towards the self may materialize. Thus, it is suggested here that when a person has realistic aspirations or expectations and is prepared to work to achieve those aspirations, then success in their endeavours can contribute towards a positive attitude and belief in oneself.

Individual differences as buffers against stressors

One question here is whether some people are more prone to the effects of stressors and others are not? A very early and classic study (Kobasa, Hilker and Maddi, 1979) explored personality traits in highly stressed executives in a number of occupations. Those participants who reported less illness in their lives showed three kinds of protective traits that they termed 'hardiness'. These protective traits were: (1) an openness to change, (2) feeling committed and involved and (3) feeling in control over their lives. The most important of these was the participants 'openness to change'. It seemed that those who were open to change interpreted future events to their advantage and this reduced their levels of stress and the overall effects of the stressor on the person.

For example, how do people react when a major business closes and people are laid off from their work? All of those affected will interpret this event as a major change in their lives and it has the potential to be major stressor that moves around future financial security for the person and their family. Usually, when a business closes the workers are each offered a financial settlement or a redundancy payment. In the short term the benefits of a large amount of money may seem like a financial windfall. However, once the redundancy is spent or used up some people could develop a negative attitude about the future. It is possible that they will view the future prospects as including: (1) limited chances of getting a job due to competition from colleagues, (2) being less financially sound, (3) having to live below previous standards and (4) the possibility of increasing debts. Certainly, when the situation is viewed from this perspective, the future does look bleak.

The person who is not open to change is more likely to see the job loss as a demoralizing event and is very likely to suffer the negative physiological and psychological effects of this stressor. In such people, being unemployed for a lengthy period of time and having no opportunity of a job could signal the onset of hopelessness about job prospects in the future. Couple this with a decrease in living standards and you have the basic ingredients for additional psychosocial stressors, crisis and possible suicide-related behaviour in the future. However, other people may see the loss of their job as a challenge for the future. They may decide on how to use their redundancy payment to their best advantage and invest in a chance to develop a new career that is better suited to their abilities.

In doing so, they will consider various options all of which will have the potential for future financial security for them and their family. Of course in new ventures nothing can be guaranteed but if they take on board advice given from reputable sources, then the future could be brighter.

The person's behavioural response to crisis

Whenever the person reaches a crisis point they have to make a decision that will somehow deal with the stressor. This decision could include a want to live or a want to die on the part of the person. Unfortunately, how the person makes the decision to live or die is not usually that clear cut. As mentioned earlier, many self-harm acts started when a person first tried to kill him or herself. For example, take Case vignette 4 where Stephen was admitted to accident and emergency after taking an overdose of paracetamol. Analysis of his suicidal intention suggested that he did try to kill himself. Indeed, he even admitted such in his interview. However, he survived and after brief crisis intervention counselling he returned home where he had support from both family and friends. In this scenario, Stephen makes a decision to live after he had survived an attempt to kill himself. However, Sarah in Case vignette 3 gives a different interpretation of the want to live. Initially Sarah commenced her self-harm behaviour by wanting to kill herself. Her story reveals that she did find solace in abusing alcohol and in taking overdoses. In addition, Marie in Case vignette 2 shows that she did not care whether she lived or died. In fact, in her first cutting episode she wanted more to die than she did to live. However, she got so much relief out of her cutting on the first time that she used cutting on other occasions as a means of relieving her despair and curtailing her suicide thoughts.

Case vignettes 2, 3 and 4 are not academic proof that all those people who self-harm have initially attempted suicide. However, these vignettes do serve the purpose to make the point that some people who self-harm started from a premise of wanting to die but then moved to a position of wanting to live. In doing so, it has got to be acknowledged that many people who self-harm do so as a means of coping with their emotional turmoil and as a means of preventing their own suicide. In other words, self-harm is one way that people use to prevent their own suicide (NICE, 2004a; Pembroke, 1998a). Thus, as outlined in Figure 3.1 and in Figure 5.1, when a person chooses self-harm as a response to stressors in their lives, they have chosen a life option.

On the other hand, the person may choose a death option as a response to crisis. At this point, the person is suffering severe emotional turmoil or psychache (Shneidman, 1993). Analysis of people's behaviour prior to their suicide indicates that in most cases there were warning signs. Frequently these signs are verbal in that the person says something that sounds out of place. For instance, 'It's not worth it any more.' Or 'What's the sense of going on, life's a drag.' These verbal signs may have been given to someone such as a member of the family, a friend, or a work colleague. In addition, these verbal signals can be mentioned at any time and in any place. From an anecdotal point of view a female friend of mine once had a conversation at a midnight beach party when a friend of hers talked about having thoughts of suicide. Also, another friend of mine told me that he was on a taxi journey when the taxi driver started to talk to him about his suicidal thoughts. In addition, I had a similar personal experience one day while I was out fishing along the riverbank when a friend started to talk about his suicidal thoughts. These anecdotal examples may seem strange but they are true and they serve to point out that some people do give signals and they also seek help when considering suicide-related behaviour.

In addition, when a person has decided that they are going to kill themselves they may give the appearance of settling their business affairs in preparation for their planned death. For instance, as mentioned earlier, some people may settle financial matters and make a will. Sometimes they give away valuables and personal belongings. This latter behaviour may be accompanied by the statement that they don't need them any more or words to that effect. Another warning sign that may suggest that the person is considering suicide is some behaviour that appears out of the ordinary or not usual for the person. More often than not the person may appear as if they have lost interest in their appearance and they might limit their interaction with others. They may have a disturbed sleep pattern and have recently begun to look tired or dishevelled. In contrast, Shea (2002) points out that some people who have made up their mind to kill themselves suddenly become very calm. It is as if they know that their psychache will soon end. For example, see Case vignette 23.

Case vignette 23

As a very junior student I can recall a very quiet and gentle person whom I shall call Martin. He was in his mid-forties and he had spent most of his adult life in a psychiatric hospital. He had a long history of clinical depression and to some degree had become institutionalized and very dependant on the hospital. He had always resisted any help from practitioners that tried to rehabilitate him or would give him some degree of freedom outside of the hospital. He was difficult to motivate and seemed totally uninterested in most things that were going on around him. He was the last to get up out of bed in the mornings and even though he had a part-time job helping with the delivery service in the hospital, it was difficult to get him to start on time. At mealtimes, Martin always played with his food and he was the last to leave the table. Generally speaking he took no interest in any other activities, nor did he show any interest in interacting with other people in the ward setting.

I can vividly recall the last day that I saw Martin alive. It was a beautiful sunny day and Martin was the first out of bed. He had a spring in his step and he finished his breakfast like I never saw before. He was talkative and happy. All of the staff noticed this and everyone was so happy about it. It was so nice to see Martin smile and talk to other people. After breakfast, he waited outside the ward for the delivery van to arrive for him. This was a first and the van driver even commented on it. Martin just smiled. At dinnertime Martin came back to the ward and had his meal and asked for a second helping. In addition, he was jovial with everyone there. Later in the evening, he had his tea and said he was going for a walk. However, he never returned. Martin had gone and sat on a railway track and waited for a particular train that was usually on time. Just before I went off duty, the ward manager was asked to go and help identify Martin's remains.

I had known Martin for some time before he killed himself. He was a familiar sight on the delivery van and he never missed a day of his work. However, he always gave me the impression of a deeply troubled man. I did try to talk to him on a number of occasions but his responses were always brief and did not invite friendly conversation. I noticed that he responded similarly to other staff as well. Martin gave the impression that he did not want to communicate with other people. When I reflected on the events that occurred on the day that he died, I realized that there was a great calmness about him. It was as if he had made up his mind and that he could see that the end of his emotional despair was near. In a way the short story by Edgor Allen Poe 'A Descent into the Maelström' (Galloway, 1967) is very appropriate. The man in the story is staring into the depths of the maelstrom (whirlpool) and knows that there is nothing that he or his brother can do but accept their fate. I have always come to the conclusion that Martin had made a very firm decision to die and once made he totally accepted his fate. While some practitioners might judge whether or not Martin's suicide was right or wrong or whether it was rational or irrational; there is the possibility that Martin may have come to the conclusion that his suicide was the right or rational answer to his own personal psychache. Unfortunately we will never know the answer to this as Martin did not leave a suicide note nor did he give any explanation for his unusual, but very welcome, behaviour during his last day alive.

Discussion points: In a small group (no more than six students) spend 10–15 minutes discussing Case vignette 23. What would you do if you noticed unusual behavioural changes in one of your friends or one of your work colleagues? Write down some notes on your decisions and compare these notes with other groups. Make sure that you include rationale for your decisions.

Help-seeking behaviour – contact with the caring services

According to the pathways in Figure 3.1, a person can seek help at any time and not necessarily only when they are in crisis. Furthermore, it has long been known that many people will communicate their thoughts before suicide-related behaviour (Hawton and Blackstock, 1976; Bancroft *et al.*, 1977; Turner, 1982; Brent *et al.*, 1988; Diekstra and Van Egmond, 1989; Vassilas and Morgan, 1993; Stenager and Jensen, 1994; Cheng, 1995; Handwerk *et al.*, 1998; Samaritans, 2006; LivingWorks, 2004). Some studies report that those who tried to kill themselves had sought help in the month prior to their suicide attempt (Crockett, 1987; van Casteren *et al.*, 1993; Stenager and Jensen, 1994; DoH, 2001). However, almost 50% of clients, after consulting with their GP, used the prescribed medicine for a suicide-related behaviour (Crockett, 1987; Stenager and Jensen, 1994; Ohberg *et al.*, 1996).

Discussion points: In a small group (no more than six students) spend 10–15 minutes discussing how you would feel if you had to talk to your GP or other practitioner about a very personal issue that was causing you distress. Write down some notes on your decisions and compare these notes with other groups. Make sure that you include rationale for your decisions.

In addition, some early researchers reported that while most had made contact with their GP, only about 25% had contacted the psychiatric services (Bancroft *et al.*, 1977). Also, they reported that while 18% had asked for psychiatric help, some 55% of individuals said that they had wanted 'someone to talk to'. It is worth noting that most of those who killed themselves, while contacting their GPs prior to their suicide, did not contact the psychiatric services. It seems that many of those who died by suicide did not acknowledge their psychological symptoms to their GP, preferring to focus on physical symptoms and physical health needs (Clark and Fawcett, 1992). Other researchers suggest that those aged under 35 might not think it appropriate to discuss emotional or psychological problems with a doctor (Vassilas and Morgan, 1993).

In more recent times, it has been reported that almost 20% of those who killed themselves made contact in the 24 hours prior to their suicide and that 48% had made contact with caring professionals in the week preceding their suicide (DoH, 2001). Most of these contacts were face to face with a consultant, junior psychiatrist or a mental health nurse. Furthermore, in 70% of cases the contact was routine rather than urgent. In almost half of these suicides, the person's key worker was in attendance at the meeting (DoH, 2001).

Some early studies suggested that many young people do not consult their GP because they perceive them as having disapproving attitudes, or as being unsympathetic or too busy to help them (Hawton and Blackstock, 1976) and many young people are suspicious of statutory services (Woods, 1990). It has also been reported that many young people did not know where to go if they wanted to talk to someone about themselves or their relationships (Homefirst Community Trust, 1997). Also, McGonagle and Gentle (1996) found that clients with enduring mental illness failed to attend a day hospital because of a lack of partnerships in decisions on choice of therapy, lack of individualized care, and not being listened to. These findings echo Evans, Cox and Turnball (1992) who reported that those clients who self-harmed perceived that their views were not listened to and that help from some practitioners was useless. Even in more recent times, Dorer *et al.* (1999) suggested that in general, adolescents expect to be judged harshly and to be told off for wasting staff time. Following these reports, one would have expected that practitioners' attitudes to young people who self-harm would improve; however the Mental Health Foundation and the Camelot Foundation report that these negative attitudes are still in evidence (MHF/CF, 2006).

Boldero and Fallon (1995) found that adolescents' help-seeking behaviour was determined by an interplay of factors including sex, age and type of problem. Also, adolescents have ideas about the suitability of professional helpers. For example, friends were asked for help in interpersonal difficulties, teachers were consulted for education difficulties, and other professionals for health difficulties (Conrad, 1991). Similarly, Boldero and Fallon (1995) reported that young people do seek help for life's difficulties but not always from practitioners nor from family. The reliance on friends for help in interpersonal difficulties is worth noting, bearing in mind the high incidence of self-harm as a result of interpersonal difficulties (Conrad, 1992; Hawton *et al.*, 2000). In addition, adolescents can be influenced by the suicidal death of a friend and clustering of suicides can occur (Turano, 1996). Furthermore, the recent report by the Institute of Public Policy research (IPPR, 2006) maintains that British adolescents spend more time in the company of their peers and less time with adults and parents than children from other countries. While social support networks and especially friendships are very necessary, one has to wonder how immature adolescents would respond to peers who are very emotionally upset.

Early authors suggested that people who self-harmed had different character-istics to those who contacted the Samaritans and that while listening to the person in distress, the Samaritans could do very little in the way of prevention (Kreitman and Chowdhury, 1973). Also, it was reported that few people who self-harmed had contacted the Samaritans prior to the behaviour (Bancroft *et al.*, 1977). However, Ray (1996, p. 7) asserts that callers to the Samaritans 'retain the ultimate control over their lives, while still having access to emotional support'. Also, in more recent times the Samaritans (2006) report that in as many as 20% of the calls they receive the person expresses suicidal thoughts and there are many calls from people who regularly self-harm. Currently there is a need to update Kreitman and Chowdhury's (1973) work.

In more recent times, it appears that the response by practitioners to those admitted following suicide-related behaviour is mixed. There is still evidence of people, particularly those in care after an episode of self-harm, experiencing negative responses from health carers (Harris, 2000; Jeffrey and Warm, 2002) and still experiencing frustration about their care in hospital (Smith, 2002). The perception was that staff did not understand and saw them as failures. This is similar to the findings reported by Castillo, Allen and Coxhead (2001). In Harris's (2000) study, it seems that practitioners actually told female participants that they were time wasting. In contrast to all the negative reports in the past, some recent authors suggest that adolescents' experiences of health care are becoming more positive. For example, Dorer *et al.* (1999) report that almost half of their sample (n = 43) was positive about their hospital experience. In this report health care staff were cited as being friendly and non-judgemental. They (Dorer *et al.*, 1999, p. 415) also reported that adolescents' experiences of hospital were 'a chance to rest and think things through with the pressures removed, and meeting other young people – some of whom had also taken an overdose'. Other authors such as Burgess, Hawton and Loveday (1998) had previously reported similar findings. Thus, there is a hint that, in some cases, practitioners' responses to self-harm and to those who attempt suicide is improving. If, in a general sense, this is the case, it is a major leap forward in the type of care required by those contemplating or after having carried out self-harm behaviour or those who survived an attempt at suicide. However, Dorer *et al.* (1999) suggest that those who did not participate in the study may have had different experiences. Therefore, these findings, while offering some support for practitioners' interventions, need to be treated with caution. Nonetheless, even though there are difficulties in recruiting participants, additional research is still warranted in ascertaining the person's experience of care. This information is very necessary in order for practitioners to improve the care they provide.

Making contact with another human being and opening up to them about one's own very personal and very private difficulties is a very important step. The literature suggests that those with psychache and in need of psychological help value friendly and non-judgemental responses (Burgess, Hawton and Loveday, 1998; Dorer *et al.*, 1999; Smith, 2002; Lindgren *et al.*, 2004). This applies equally whether the help is sought from professional health carers or from non-professional people like family, friends or other individuals. How a person communicates their difficulties is important. As stated previously, their communications to practitioners may be vague and relate to physical difficulties (Chin, Touquet and Burns, 1986; Clark and Fawcett, 1992; DoH, 2001) rather than focusing on their psychological difficulties. Males certainly have a difficulty is talking about their psychological difficulties. Indeed males may not seek help at all. This is dangerous as not communicating about one's psychological difficulties or having a low number of communications can pre-empt suicide (Handwerk *et al.*, 1998).

Assuming that help was sought by the person and that they received that help and that issues had been dealt with, then the stressor would have been resolved or the physical and psychological effects of the stressor would have been reduced. Carlton and Deane (2000) suggest that when adolescents have previously received help in a crisis situation, this can result in higher intentions to seek help in the future should their thoughts turn to suicide. However, irrespective of whether the person talks openly or very directly about their difficulties to others or whether the person vaguely talks about their difficulties to others, the perceived reception that they get from family, friends or health care practitioners is important. For example, if the person believes that help is not forthcoming, their evaluation of their attempts to resolve their stressor to date may turn their thoughts and ideas to more radical behavioural responses. These responses, while not excluding a wide range of other behaviours to help minimize or reduce the effects of the stressors, may include suicide-related behaviour.

Stressor resolved

As viewed in Figure 3.1, the person's initial response to the stressor or potential stressor involves both physiological (central nervous system) and psychological responses (other coping mechanisms). Both sets of responses have important roles to play in preparing and protecting the person from the effects of the stressor. If the person's coping mechanism moderates the effects of the stressors or better still resolves issues that brought the stressor to the fore, then the body will quickly return to its pre-stress levels. The parasympathetic nervous system will relax the effects of the sympathetic nervous system. This action by the parasympathetic nervous system will bring about almost immediate relief and allow the person to relax. Along with this, the person's psychological coping mechanism may be internalized and may be used in any similar stress-invoking situation in the future. In brief, the person can learn from any experience that allowed them to problem-solve or come to terms with their difficulties.

Stressor unresolved – crisis

However, Figure 3.1 also shows that should the person's physical and psychological responses fail to resolve, reduce or moderate the effects of the stressor, the person's psychological and biological reserves will be called upon. It is important to remember that these physical effects of stress are the same as those experienced, by any person, during periods of anxiety. However, when the stressor is unresolved after attempts at resolution, the physical effects will increase in intensity during the resistance stage (Selye, 1956). Practitioners, who have experienced the physical effects of anxiety during their own lives, should be able to relate to what it must be like when these feelings are intensified. In addition, the person's psychological attempts at resolving the stressor, including some form of communication with others, may have been ineffective. Failure in these forms of communication can compound the physical effects with resultant negative thoughts about one's ability to obtain help in resolving the stressor. A failure to moderate or resolve the stressor at this stage can lead to the exhaustion stage (Selye, 1956).

In the exhaustion stage the person's biological and psychological reserves have become depleted or are near to doing so. In effect, the person is in great need of both physiological and psychological help. Even if help is available but is perceived by the person as being, for whatever reason, unobtainable then helplessness can occur (Seligman, 1975; Miller, 1980) and even hopelessness about the future can develop (Beck *et al.*, 1974, 1985, 1993; Beck, Kovacs and Weissman, 1975; Morano, Cisler and Lemerond, 1993; MacLeod, Rose and Williams, 1993; Hawton, 1994b; Mendonca and Holden, 1996; McLaughlin, Miller and Warwick, 1996; Lindgren *et al.*, 2004). In turn these thoughts can increase the intensity of the psychache and eventually lead to a crisis situation in the person's life. Even at the stage of crisis, as seen in Figure 3.1, the possibility of resolving the stressor that has led to this intensified distress still exists. If appropriate help is offered, given and accepted, the person should be able to access that healing route in the left hand column of Figure 3.1. On the other hand, the person may, due to their emotional state, not be able to access potential help. Quite possibly the person may be physically weak or psychologically unable to help himself or even seek help from others. Practitioners will be able to make links between psychache and clinical terms such as low self-esteem, withdrawn, depression, anxiety, helplessness, hopelessness and crisis. If a person is experiencing or demonstrating signs of these, then suicide-related behaviour may be chosen as a way of dealing with the stressor.

For many people experiencing despair or psychache, the thought of suicide may be their response. However, whether they choose to act on their thoughts and die by suicide will depend on their rationale for dying. As mentioned earlier, approximately 24% of people who present at accident and emergency for the first time will repeat the behaviour (Zahl and Hawton, 2004) at some stage in the future. Of the 24% of people who repeat the behaviour, many will use some form of self-harm as a coping mechanism for their despair. Unfortunately, it is acknowledged that many of those who repeat the behaviour or who repetitively use self-harm will eventually kill themselves (DHSSPSNI, 2006). Therefore, the risk of future suicide will need to be assessed in all those people who survive a suicide attempt.

Summary

In this chapter some of the person's responses to crisis and to issues that are causing them severe emotional despair or psychache have been outlined. The biological effects of distress on the person can exacerbate the person's feelings of despair and their cognitive and behavioural responses to the stressor. The increased effects of the sympathetic nervous system, which creates all the symptoms of anxiety, may be calmed if the stressor is resolved and the parasympathetic nervous system becomes operationalized. However, while anxioltic medication can settle the effects of the sympathetic nervous system, it cannot resolve the issues that are causing distress or despair in the person. Also, if the stressor is not resolved and if the effects of the sympathetic nervous system are not reduced then the person's anxiety will increase and (s)he may enter into a state of emotional distress.

Alternatively, when some people come to a crisis point, they can think about suicide or they can then transform their thoughts about suicide into a more positive attitude about the future. For instance, some people can call on their psychological coping skills and in particular their problem-solving skills to resolve their crisis. When distressing situations are known about in advance then the person may be able to practise in preparation for dealing with the potential stressor. Other people may take up some physical exercise in an effort to minimize the feelings associated with emotional distress. Social support in the form of friends and family is also very useful and is an important buffer against emotional despair and possible suicide-related behaviour. In addition, a person may respond in other ways. For example, they may have a positive attitude towards life in general. Even though they have experienced great despair, their own positive attitude towards themselves may prevent them from moving towards suicide-related behaviour. From a behavioural point of view, some people do contemplate and carry out suicide-related behaviour. First, it can be quite difficult to tell if a person is self-harming until it has been brought to the attention of family, friends, or medical personnel. Quite a few people do manage to hide, for a lengthy period of time, their distress, emotional despair and their self-harming behaviour away from others. More often than not others only know about it when the person is admitted to hospital. Second, it is well known about that most people will give verbal and behavioural warning signs prior to their suicide. Some of these signs may be very subtle and others more glaring. However, it is incumbent on practitioners to notice these signs and help the person begin the process of healing or easing their psychache.

Caring responses to suicide-related behaviour

7

As mentioned earlier, stressors that create emotional distress and that are linked to suicide-related behaviour can emanate from any number of sources. While some of these sources may be linked to the client's inner self, some stressors may come from outside of the client's physical self and will be environmental or situational in nature. Frequently the client may perceive these sources as being outside of their control. Gaining control of a stressful situation or event is easier said than done and more often than not there is no one response that will uniformly fix all forms of stressors that lead to suicide-related behaviour within people. In the following chapters the main concern is to explore how practitioners can respond in a caring and therapeutic way to those experiencing psychache. In this chapter we will explore issues involved in providing a caring response to clients who are experiencing psychache or crisis and when suicide-related behaviour has become an option. Also, an example of a caring response to suicide-related behaviour is given in order to generate discussion among readers. The following issues are specifically addressed in this chapter:

1. The case for a caring response
2. Personal qualities of the practitioner
   (a) Self-awareness
   (b) Confidentiality
   (c) Unconditional positive regard
   (d) Congruence
   (e) Empathy

3. The skills required in the therapeutic relationship

    (a) Non-verbal cues as a means of communicating

    (b) Verbal responses in the therapeutic relationship

    (c) Paraphrasing in the therapeutic relationship

    (d) Reflection in the therapeutic relationship

    (e) Questions in the therapeutic relationship

    (f) Silence in the therapeutic relationship

4. An example of a caring response

The case for a caring response

Caring is an essential component in the ethos of all health care practitioners. Yet there are difficulties in defining what constitutes caring. Most early studies come from a nursing background and suggest that caring involves having a positive attitude towards clients and being competent in practice. However, Wolf (1986) reported that 'attentive listening', 'honesty' and 'patience' were also important qualities in defining caring. In addition, Morrison (1990) also reported that psychological factors were important. Therefore, from a mental health point of view a caring response need not necessarily be a physical response and indeed would include spending appropriate time with clients, actively listening to them and even helping them work through an emotional crisis. We are aware that many people who are experiencing suicide-related behaviour will subtly give both verbal and behavioural signals in advance (LivingWorks, 2004). These signals can occur at any time and in any place but an astute family member, friend or practitioner may be able to tune into them. It is thus not surprising to know that a caring response to those experiencing suicide-related behaviour may be required in any location and in any situation. For example, while most practitioners would indicate the hospital ward as the main place of care, anecdotal evidence indicates that other places may be used: (1) in a person's home; (2) in the pub; (3) on the river bank; or even (4) in a taxi. Also, it is well known that self-harm indicates deep anguish within a person and that it is a major indicator of future suicide. While some signals are subtle, self-harm or attempted suicide, when it comes to the attention of family, friends or practitioners, is a signal that is loud and clear. Therefore, a key component in a caring response is that practitioners recognize and acknowledges a person's signals of despair or crisis and respond to them. These signals are really invitations to engage with the person and for practitioners not to take these signals seriously may actually contribute towards a number of suicides.

    Discussion points: In a small group (no more than six students) spend 10–15 minutes to (1) draw up a list of the types of names or comments that you have heard from practitioners when referring to people who self-harm and (2) make notes on the ways you have seen practitioners respond to people who have a previous history of self-harm. When you have finalized your lists you should then compare your notes with those in other groups.

So what is the health care response to the possibility of suicide-related behaviour within the supposedly safe environs of its hospitals? More often than not the focus is on the safety of its inpatients. The DoH (2001) recommended that clients who are at risk of suicide should be constantly observed. In recent times such observations have been called 'close observation', 'special observation' and 'constant observation'. However, such observation practices have come under criticism. For example, Bowers, Gournay and Duffy (2000) reported that national guidelines for this practice did not exist: others report observational practices as being less than therapeutic (Whittington and McLaughlin, 2000; Bowles et al., 2002); or not being practised as planned (Neilson and Brennan, 2001). There are inherent difficulties in the implementation of such observation policies and Duffy (1995) pointed out that while they contained features that were controlling they also had features that offered the possibility of helping as well. Unfortunately, much of the research suggests that staff did not avail themselves of the caring or helping opportunities that were possible in special observation. Duffy (1995) also pointed out that the non-therapeutic nature of the care resulted from a custodial, paternalistic and medical model of care. In addition, the Sainsbury Centre for Mental Health (SCMH, 1998, 2002) has made a number of recommendations regarding improving the therapeutic nature of acute wards.

Certainly, the viewpoint as outlined above suggests that there is a great need to improve the delivery of care in the acute mental health setting. It is well known that suicide-related behaviour is a multi-faceted phenomenon and it will therefore require a multi-faceted response from practitioners. What does seem to be coming through is that in many cases, practitioners are willing to do more but are restricted in so doing due to operational and managerial policies. While custodial care and observational practices have not diminished the number of inpatient suicides (DoH, 2001), other authors make the point that engagement with clients may provide a genuine alternative to observation schedules (Bowles et al., 2002). What is needed in the acute admission wards is that practitioners need to ring fence the time they spend with their clients. For instance, regarding mental health nursing Peplau (1994) makes it very clear that each nurse should allocate specific time every working day for each of the clients that they are responsible for. This time must include one-to-one interaction where the nurse engages with the client regarding the client's psychological care needs.

A number of reports suggest that just being with clients and also communicating with them about their suicide-related behaviour is very helpful (McLaughlin, 1999; Whittington and McLaughlin, 2000; Dunne, Thompson and

Leitch, 2000; Samuelsson *et al.*, 2000; Bowles *et al.*, 2002; Lindgren *et al.*, 2004). However, there is sometimes the belief that talking to clients about suicide-related behaviour could instigate suicidal thinking in clients. This is not the case and this point is made very well in the Applied Suicide Intervention Skills Training (LivingWorks, 2004). When a practitioner thinks that a client is considering suicide-related behaviour, then it would be most appropriate for them to ask outright about it. For instance, they could say to such a client 'Are you thinking about killing yourself? ' This type of direct question shows that the practitioner is not afraid, is interested and is willing to talk. Also, it might be the spur to allow the client to talk openly and begin to tell their story. If the client confirms that they are thinking about suicide-related behaviour, then a connection has been made between the client and the practitioner. Here, the practitioner is being given an opportunity to establish what is known as a therapeutic relationship with the client. At this point, they need not be a qualified counsellor/psychotherapist but they should exhibit certain professional qualities. These qualities will now be explored.

Personal qualities of the practitioner

When responding to the emotional needs of a fellow human being, all practitioners must first know what it is to be human. Indeed, theorists and practitioners alike will agree that all practitioners must be able to answer the questions 'Who am I?' and 'What is it like to be me?' These questions may, to the uninitiated, seem to be philosophical. However, they do ask the practitioners to understand themselves first before they try to understand others. The extent to which a practitioner can answer the questions could impinge on the quality of the relationship between the client and the practitioner.

Discussion points: In a small group (no more than six students) spend 10–15 minutes discussing (i) how you would feel if you had to discuss your personal (emotional) issues with a practitioner and (ii) if you were to draw up a list of qualities that the practitioner must exhibit before you would talk to him or her, what would it include? Begin each quality with the words, 'The practitioner must be able to demonstrate . . .' When you have finalized your list you should then write a rationale for each quality and compare these notes with other groups.

What criteria should a practitioner have within their psyche? Some of the founding fathers of interpersonal relationships made profound comments, which are still valuable today. For instance, Peplau (1952) was the first to coin the phrase 'nurse–patient relationship'. Her theory of psychodynamic nursing was well before its time and is still as valid now as it was over 50 years ago. In fact, for over 40 years she published on a regular basis and remained as passionate about the importance of the nurse–patient relationship as ever. Another eminent interaction theory at that time was proposed by Rogers (1951, 1961). He posited the thought that if he could produce a certain type of relationship, then the client would be able to discover within him or herself the ability to grow, change and foster personal development. Currently, many textbooks on health care will mention what is needed to form a therapeutic relationship between practitioners and clients. The problem is whether or not some readers actually analyse and take on board or internalize the issues involved in the therapeutic relationship. Can they measure up? First of all, you should look at the qualities that your group discussion raised in the above activity. Each of you will be the future practitioner. Will you measure up to the qualities that your group has proposed? Let's explore some of the qualities that appear in the literature and that your group may have raised.

(a) Self-awareness

This is a key component in the helping arsenal of the practitioner. In order to help people in psychological distress or despair, all practitioners must be able to draw on their own personal experience of emotions such as happiness, sadness, anxiety, fear, frustration and anger. Also, practitioners must be able to explore and examine their own responses to such emotions. One model of exploring the self is the Johari window as described by Luft and Ingham (1963). In brief, this window contains four quadrants, which are:

1. **Open self:** This quadrant contains those personal details that you and others know about you. In this area you will have no problem sharing information about yourself with others. This quadrant will increase in size as you gain trust in others.

2. **Blind self:** This quadrant is a part of you that you don't see and are unaware of. It is like the back of your head, everyone else can see it but you can't. However, you can see it with a mirror. In a caring situation, the mirror will be the practitioner. This quadrant contains blind spots and these can be positive and negative. Sometimes you will irritate others and the blind spot is that you don't know that you are doing it. When it is mirrored back to you (or pointed out) you become aware and need to do something about it. In contrast, some clients see only their negative side and just cannot see what is positive in their lives. Practitioners can facilitate a client to recognize these positive qualities and do something constructive with them.

3. **Hidden self:** In this quadrant you will have issues that you don't want to share with others. These are private issues that may be embarrassing or

hurtful and contain elements of guilt and shame. In an effort to maintain our dignity a person will put on a façade. More often than not, therapy encourages self-disclosure and a reduction in the size of the area in this quadrant.

4. **Unknown self:** In this quadrant there are issues that neither you nor anyone else is aware of. As they are in the subconscious it is difficult for you and others to access them. In the unknown area you could have unrecognized learning resources and opportunities. Frequently, discussion in caring situations can produce some unexpected insights into unknown strengths.

The aim of self-awareness is to increase the area of the 'open self' quadrant and to decrease the size of the area in each of the other three quadrants. For example, the practitioner can become very self-aware when they explore their own 'blind spots', 'hidden selves (facades)' and 'unknown selves' with a colleague. If embarked upon, this type of exercise would involve the practitioner self-disclosing and revealing to others very personal details about him or herself. Being able to openly discuss a personal issue with a colleague or another person will increase the area size of the 'open self' and reduce the area size of one or all three of the other quadrants. By genuinely doing so, the practitioner will experience what it is like to be in the position of a client requiring a human response to their emotional/ psychological crisis. All practitioner-training programmes will at some point refer to self-awareness and will discuss the importance of this. However, very few health care programmes actually encourage students to participate in personal therapy where they would self-disclose to others about events or issues that caused them personal distress in their lives. Rogers (1951) makes the point that personal therapy for trainees is of 'markedly significant benefit'. Unfortunately most students involved in mental health care will have little or no experience of what it is like to be in the position of a client. While Rogers (1951) made the point that personal therapy is useful for trainees; maybe its inclusion in future mental health training programmes should be evaluated.

(b) Confidentiality

This is central to the development of a trusting relationship between the practitioner and the client who requires therapy. Recently, the report of an inquiry into self-harm in young people by the Mental Health Foundation and the Camelot Foundation (MHF/CF, 2006) reported that breech of confidentiality was a major area of concern for both clients and practitioners. However, confidentiality as an entity contains both ethical and legal challenges. All professions involved in mental health care include a section on confidentiality in their Code of Conduct.

Likewise, government laws also address the degree of confidentiality as used in therapy. This seems like a double-edged sword and as such each practitioner must seriously consider the amount of confidentiality that can be allowed in a therapeutic relationship with a client. It is well recognized that true therapy cannot take place unless a client can trust what they reveal in therapy to the practitioner. Therefore, it is the responsibility of the practitioner to discuss openly with the client issues about confidentiality early in the therapeutic relationship.

In some professions such as counselling and psychotherapy, clinical supervision is mandatory for each practitioner. However, most mental health care professions will advocate the use of clinical supervisors rather than impose a mandatory ruling. This situation is open to change in the future. Nonetheless, practitioners will discuss some details about their interactions and relationships with people in their care with colleagues and with clinical supervisors. Thus, confidentiality cannot be guaranteed as being absolute. It follows that a client requiring therapy has a right to know that some of their personal details will be discussed with other practitioners. Furthermore, confidentiality must be broken when it is clear that the client is intent on harming him or herself or harming others. Also, confidentiality must be broken when child abuse, abuse of dependent adults and abuse of the elderly becomes apparent. Shea (2002) makes it clear that on some occasions the client's safety (and the safety of others) has a higher priority than confidentiality. In addition, the courts can legally request confidential information about a client if it becomes an issue in a court case.

On the whole, in the therapeutic relationship, all practitioners are duty bound to protect the information that is confided to them in therapy. As stated earlier this is a very central part of the relationship between the client and the practitioner. However, the practitioner must be honest, up front and explain to the client that the practitioner will, in general, strive to keep what is revealed in therapy confidential. However, it is best practice to discuss with the client the limitations of confidentiality as well. Corey (2005) makes the point that discussing confidential issues early in the therapeutic relationship does not necessarily impinge on the success of therapy.

(c) Unconditional positive regard

This is a very important attitude that practitioners must communicate towards their clients. In Rogers (1951) influential manuscript he used the term 'acceptance'. The client is viewed with dignity and valued as a worthwhile and positive human being. The emphasis on this attitude is that there are no conditions attached to the relationship or to the caring. In effect there are no ifs or buts to this criteria: the practitioner must accept the client as a person. For instance, practitioners cannot have the attitude of 'I will only care for you if . . .' Or another unacceptable negative attitude would be 'I would accept you but you . . .' There is no judgement or evaluation of the client and it is a case of accepting the client the way (s)he is. Most practitioners would have heard of the term 'non-judgemental'. This means that they accept that the client has his/her own beliefs and emotions and is free to express them in therapy. However, it does not mean that the practitioner condones, accepts or approves of any current or previous actions or behaviour in the client's history. While it is generally accepted that most practitioners have very positive attitudes towards clients, it is well known that negative attitudes towards clients do exist in some health carers. Attitudes such as these in persons charged with the responsibility of mental health care cannot be condoned and need to be addressed. If it is that health carers are disrespectful towards clients or that they disapprove of or dislike them, then the therapeutic relationship will not even get off the ground. In such cases health carers will need to evaluate the impact their judgemental attitude would have on clients.

(d) Congruence

In the therapeutic relationship, congruence, which some theorists call genuineness, is also an attitude recommended by Rogers (1951). By being congruent, the practitioner must exhibit genuineness at being in the relationship and that (s)he is presenting as a person who is genuinely interested in the client's story. The practitioner appears as being authentic and does not present as someone with a false face or a façade. In effect the practitioner accepts the client for who they are. Also, by being genuine the practitioner can openly express thoughts, feelings and attitudes that appear during the course of a therapeutic relationship. However, when practitioners try too hard to be genuine it can send out conflicting non-verbal communication signals and this can create difficulties in the relationship. Also, if a practitioner does not like a client but feigns acceptance, then the therapeutic relationship will fail and therapy will be unsuccessful. In contrast, if the practitioner is genuine, without façade, and is accepting of the client, then both trust and the therapeutic relationship will be developed.

(e) Empathy

According to Goleman (2006) an American psychologist by the name of Edward Bradford Titchener (1867–1927) used the term 'motor mimicry' as an original sense of the word 'empathy'. In brief, Titchener's theory of empathy came from an imitation of another's distress, which provokes similar feelings in the observer. The term itself comes from the Greek work *empatheia* which means 'feeling into'. As such, empathy is used by many theorists to describe the ability of one person being able to reflect the subjective experience of another person. Also, the importance of empathy is well made in Rogers (1951) theory. It is also a communication skill that is a cornerstone in the therapeutic relationship. According to Watson (2002) empathic understanding is a very important factor in determining a client's progress in therapy and as such it is a vital skill in the practitioner's toolbox.

The skill is to demonstrate an understanding of the client's experience by using active listening skills such as paraphrasing and reflection. The client will tell his/her story and express their thoughts by both verbal and non-verbal signals. The job of the practitioner is to metaphorically walk alongside the client as they tell their story by demonstrating their understanding of the client's experience and feelings. This must be done in an accurate and sensitive manner in a way that shows the client that the practitioner has heard and analysed what they have communicated. Being able to demonstrate accurate empathic understanding to a client also enables clients to self-disclose more about themselves (Miller, Berg and Archer, 1983).

However, being empathic is not just about demonstrating verbal skills such as paraphrasing and reflection or just about the inclusion of non-verbal body language. It is very far from being a passive activity and is very much an active interaction between the practitioner and the client. The practitioner's entire way of being must demonstrate that (s)he cares deeply about the client. In effect, they must feel the client's pain. Corey (2005) makes the point that empathy is not a skill that practitioners can call on whenever necessary but is a subjective understanding of the client with the client. In this he is indicating that practitioners, whilst operating with the client, must also maintain their own separateness. When a practitioner can grasp and show understanding of the client's world as seen by the client, and still maintain their own independence and identity, then therapy has a chance of success and the possibility of change in the client's cognitions and behaviour may occur.

The skills required in the therapeutic relationship

The practical skills involved in the therapeutic relationship include both non-verbal (body) language and verbal responses. In this book, the identified skills are briefly discussed to give the reader a basic introduction to them and to indicate their usefulness in the therapeutic relationship. However, the reader who requires more in-depth discussion on the skills would be more appropriately referred to specific texts such as Hargie and Dickson (2004), Egan (2006) or Corey (2005).

Discussion points: In a small group (no more than six students) spend 10–15 minutes carrying out the following tasks: (1) draw up a list of non-verbal signals that indicate the practitioner's interest in the client's story; (2) draw up a list of verbal responses that indicate the practitioner's interest in the client's story; (3) write down which of these two sets of skills you think is the most important; and (4) write notes on do think that your choice is more important than the other skill(s). When you have finalized drawing up your lists and writing your rationale for each set, compare your notes with those from other groups.

While some would argue that both sets of skills are of equal importance, most practitioners would agree that the way they portray themselves to clients through their body language can be more important than the verbal skills that they use. In the first instance it would be worth exploring how our non-verbal communication cues (skills) affect our interaction with others. As human beings we need people most when we are traumatized by a very serious event such as the death of a spouse or partner or when we are hospitalized due to accident or illness. It is then that most people will appreciate a visit from a friend or someone who cares. Just being there for another human being when they are facing difficulty can be very comforting for them. In the same way, being ignored by others can be very hurtful. If we can appreciate the bodily presence of a fellow human being in times of emotional distress, then we must acknowledge the effect our empathic presence can have on clients. If our physical (bodily) presence is of so much importance, then it is important that we explore how best we can use this to demonstrate our empathic presence to our clients.

(a) Non-verbal cues as a means of communicating

Our entire body is used extensively in interpersonal communication with others. Our facial expressions can indicate many of our emotions and even subtle movements of our facial muscles can send out signals to others. Sometimes, when nothing is being said, our face and body will send out signals that indicate how close or how distant the relationship is between ourselves and the client. Some of the most important skills are:

Eye contact: This is very powerful and therapeutic and shows interest. However, staring can be quite threatening. Sometimes we have to break eye contact momentarily.

Body behaviour: Our posture; how we sit; move our limbs; or make gestures with our hands.

Facial expressions: Smiles; frowns; raised eyebrows; and furrowed eyebrows. Some signals can indicate agreement, shock, horror, happiness and even anger to the client.

Proximity: This is the amount of space between ourselves and the client. Too close can be an invasion of the client's personal space and thus can be threatening. The client may interpret too great a distance as being aloof.

Tone of voice: Pitch of voice, volume, pauses, fluency and silence are all picked up on by both parties in the therapeutic relationship.

General appearance: In the same way that we look at others, so others will look at us. This issue is about the appearance of the practitioner and in particular about their grooming and their dress sense. In what way do you think a client would react to a scruffy practitioner?

Egan (2006) makes the point that attentive presence is a precursor to the client developing trust and opening up to the practitioner. He also makes the point that half-hearted presence can lead to distrust and reluctance by clients to self-disclose or share personal issues. To develop effective therapeutic relationships practitioners must be aware of the non-verbal signals they send towards clients. When we begin to become aware of our non-verbal communications, particularly in role-play situations, we can begin to address difficulties and use our non-verbal cues to enhance, rather than hinder, the therapeutic relationship. For instance SOLER is an acronym that Egan (2006) uses to outline a framework of physically tuning in to clients. However, it is not culture specific and thus may require adaptation. In brief, each letters has a particular meaning:

S: sit squarely – adopt a position that indicates you are involved with your client. When chairs are too square on, it can be seen as a threat. A slightly angled position is sometimes less threatening for the client.

O: open posture – this signals that you are open to what the client has to say. Crossing your arms may indicate defensiveness but crossing your legs may mirror the client's posture. You should evaluate the way that your posture impacts on clients.

L: lean towards the client – this signals that 'I am interested in you'. However, leaning too far forward can threaten the client's personal space, while leaning too far back can be seen as slouching and may indicate to the client that 'I am not interested in you'.

E: eye contact – this signals that 'I am interested in you'. It is not the same as staring and it should feel comfortable for both the client and you. To avoid staring, one has to look away and doing this occasionally will not breach the therapeutic relationship.

Egan (2006) makes the point that with visually impaired clients, eye contact is of no importance. However, voice direction is very important to them and they can tell from this which way the practitioner is facing. In the acronym, substitute the E for an A to become SOLAR and the A would stand for Aim. In this way visually impaired clients would know that they are being attended to.

R: relax – this is about not appearing nervous with the client. Fidgeting with your hands, moving about in your seat, or making facial expressions all indicate nervousness and can distract the client from their story. Practitioners need to control such movements.

(b) Verbal responses in the therapeutic relationship

The practitioner will also respond to clients by using a mixture of verbal skills such as paraphrasing, reflection, and asking questions. A very important point must be made at this time. In the initial stage of the therapeutic relationship, active listening is very much to the fore. It is important that the focus is on the client and that (s)he is allowed to tell their story. Poorly timed interruptions by practitioners or speaking at the same time as the client can disrupt the flow of the story. Even if the story is disjointed or told in a rushed manner, a good listener, at an appropriate time, will point these issues out to the client in a kind manner. Also, they will pick out important points in the client's story and may either paraphrase what was said or reflect on the client's emotions. For example, in the hypothetical case where Sien has poured out her story in a rush and sometimes in a disjointed way, the practitioner may respond by saying:

> Sien, you have said quite a lot there and it would be helpful for us to find out if I have understood some of the main points that you have made. For example, you said that . . .

Another skill that practitioners frequently use in their therapeutic interactions with clients is questioning. However, the difference between an interrogation and a therapeutic interaction could be defined in the way that questions are asked during the interaction. Therefore, all practitioners need to consider the appropriate use of questions in their interactions with clients. Another skill that is used, but frequently feared by practitioners in the early part of their career, is that of silence. This is a response which can appear at any time in the interaction. Also, silence has many meanings for both client and practitioner and at times there is a need to explore its meaning when it becomes apparent in the therapeutic relationship. Let's briefly explore what these skills entail and how practitioners can make use of them.

(c) Paraphrasing in the therapeutic relationship

This is a verbal skill that the practitioner uses to demonstrate that (s)he has heard and understands what the client has said. Some therapists refer to paraphrasing as a reflection of content or restatement (Hargie and Dickson, 2004). The skill involves person B (the practitioner) using his/her own words to feed back to person A (the client) what person A has just said. This skill focuses on interpreting the client's words and not on the feelings within the words. The practitioner will use similar words to those the client has used rather than use the same words. In effect, when the practitioner (person B) paraphrases what the client (person A) has just said, they are demonstrating some understanding of what the client has said. If a practitioner continually repeats words that are used by the client, then this can become frustrating for the client.

Discussion points: In a small group (no more than six students) spend 10–15 minutes discussing the following conversation between two friends who have not seen each other for a while. If you were John how would you respond to Phil's statements? Write down some notes from your discussion and compare these notes with other groups.

John: Hi Phil, long time no see. How are you and Mary?

Phil: Hi John, well I am OK but Mary and I have had an argument.

John: You and Mary have had an argument.

Phil: Aye. That's right. We went to the Night Owl Disco in Main Street and both of us got a bit drunk. You know how it is!

John: So you and Mary went to the disco and got drunk.

Phil: Aye, we did and then I went to the toilet, got sick and when I came back Joe and Mary were out slow dancing and having a snog.

John: So you went to the toilet and when you came back you found Joe and Mary having a snog on the dance floor.

Phil: That's right, I felt really angry and I went onto the dance floor and hit Joe. Then the bouncers came and threw me out. I have not heard from them since.

John: So you hit Joe and the bouncers threw you out and Joe or Mary have not spoken to you since.

Phil: Aye. That's right. Anyway, I have to go now and I will see you later.

John: OK. Phil, I will see you later. Don't worry I am sure that everything will work out with you and Mary.

In the above interaction the information that Phil provides is ripe for exploration but John misses the point. It is obvious to all and sundry that Phil feels bad about what has happened but John does not make use of the opportunity to help Phil by exploring his verbalizations or his feelings. John tends to repeat or 'parrot' only what Phil has said and demonstrates no understanding of what Phil has just told him. In addition, it would seem that Phil wanted to talk about what had happened but this was stifled by John's parroting. Paraphrasing is definitely not parroting what was said. It is about John interpreting what Phil has said and then using his own words to demonstrate to Phil that he understands what was said. Also, it is not an easy skill to develop and will require practice on the part of the keen practitioner. Such practice would involve video work with a colleague. From a training point of view it will also include constructive, and truthful, feedback on one's communication skills. The essence of paraphrasing is to demonstrate to the client that you have heard what they have said, have analysed what was said and have understood what was said. You are demonstrating to them that you are on their wavelength. The hard part of paraphrasing is to use your words, not the client's, to demonstrate your understanding of their words. Let's look at a retake of the above interaction:

> John: Hi Phil, long time no see. How are you and Mary?
> Phil: Hi John, well I am OK but Mary and I have had an argument.
> John: Oh *(feeling of surprise)*.
> Phil: Aye. That's right. We went to the Night Owl Disco in Main Street and both of us got a bit drunk. You know how it is!
> John: Mmmh.
> Phil: Aye, and then I went to the toilet, got sick and when I came back Joe and Mary were out slow dancing and having a snog.
> John: So you think that Joe moved in on Mary when you were at the toilet.
> Phil: That's right, I felt really angry and I went onto the dance floor and hit Joe. Then the bouncers came and threw me out. I have not heard from either of them since.
> John: Mmmh, so you think now that your reaction to Joe and Mary having a snog may have lost you the friendship of both and possibly your relationship with Mary?
> Phil: Aye. That's right. I don't know what is happening now and I don't know how to deal with it.
> John: OK, what about going for a cup of coffee and talking about what you might do now?
> Phil: Yea, that might be very useful. I'd appreciate that.

Discussion points: In a small group (no more than six students) spend 10–15 minutes discussing the above conversation between John and Phil who have not seen each other for a while. If you were Phil what would be your evaluation of John's responses? Write down some notes from your discussion and compare these notes with other groups.

The differences between the first and the second meetings might be worth noting. In the first meeting, John very much parrots what Phil has to say and it is quite obvious from Phil's final comment that he can't wait to get away from John. However, in the second conversation, there are two issues. Firstly, John does not judge any of Phil's activities and secondly he demonstrates some understanding of what Phil has said. This is what paraphrasing is about. It is not about parroting but about demonstrating your non-judgemental attitude and your understanding of what the client has said by reconstructing the client's words with your own.

(d) Reflection in the therapeutic relationship

In the therapeutic relationship the skill of reflection is also very important. This skill focuses on the client's emotions and it is the practitioner's responsibility to demonstrate their understanding of the client's emotions by reflecting them back to them. In doing so the practitioner acknowledges the client's feelings and their emotional pain. Additionally, reflection can encourage the client to self-disclose more about their feelings. Let's look at the conversation again:

John: Hi Phil, long time no see. How are you and Mary?
Phil: Aye John, well I am OK but Mary and I have had an argument.
John: Oh *(feeling of surprise)*.
Phil: Aye. That's right. We went to the Night Owl Disco in Main Street and both of us got a bit drunk. You know how it is!
John: Mmmh.
Phil: Aye, and then I went to the toilet, got sick and when I came back Joe and Mary were out slow dancing and having a snog.
John: So you think that Joe moved in on Mary when you were at the toilet.
Phil: That's right, I felt really angry and I went onto the dance floor and hit Joe. Then the bouncers came and threw me out. I have not heard from either of them since.
John: Mmmh, so now you feel that your reaction may have lost you the friendship of both and possibly your relationship with Mary?
Phil: Aye. That's right. I feel terrible about the whole thing. I don't know what is happening now and I don't know how to deal with it.
John: It sounds to me that you are very upset and worried about the possibility of losing the relationship with Mary and your friendship with Joe.
Phil: That's about right. I like Joe but I don't like what he did and I am really worried about losing Mary. We have been together for almost a year now.
John: Mmmh, maybe it might be helpful for you to talk about it. What about both of us going for a cup of coffee and you can talk about how you might be able to deal with it?
Phil: Yea, that might be very useful.

Both paraphrasing and reflection are skills that reflect on issues that are important to clients. Thus, paraphrasing is a form of reflection. However, the main difference between the latter two conversations is that under paraphrasing, John demonstrates some understanding of what Phil is saying. However, in reflection, as in the above conversation, John also focuses on what Phil is feeling and acknowledges his emotional pain. Both skills can thus be used very effectively to acknowledge and demonstrate understanding of issues that impinge on a client's life.

(e) Questions in the therapeutic relationship

As sociable creatures we frequently seek information about our environment and those in it. To this end, asking questions is probably one of the most widely used skills in human interactions. Questions come in many guises and Rudyard Kipling (1902) in his famous short story book, written for his children, drew attention to what is nowadays a familiar categorization:

> I keep six honest serving men,
> They taught me all I knew;
> Their names are What and Why and When,
> And How and Where and Who.

Most practitioners will be familiar with using questions in their everyday interactions with clients. Also, they will be able to relate to a number of classifications such as open questions, closed questions, recall questions, process questions, affective questions, and leading questions. A difficulty here is that many of those beginning their careers in the health care professions think that the more questions you ask, the more helpful you are. Unfortunately this is not the case. For example, I can recall a somewhat now dated film called *Uncle Buck*. In this film the late John Candy plays Uncle Buck who is asked to look after his brother's children for a few days. On the first morning he meets his nephew (played by a very young Macaulay Culkin). The ensuing interrogation of Uncle Buck by his nephew is sociably funny but in terms of a therapeutic interaction it is a perfect example of how not to ask questions. Indeed the number of closed questions that were asked within the first minute would make any practitioner squirm with embarrassment. In the therapeutic relationship, it is not the quantity of questions that is important; it is the purpose of the question that is important. For instance, practitioners should first understand why they are asking questions. This may seem like an absurd statement; however, we have to consider as to who benefits from the questions that are asked. If we consider that the therapeutic relationship is about helping the client to regain self-autonomy, then questions must benefit the client's thought processes and not just be an information-gathering session by the practitioner.

In the therapeutic relationship practitioners need to first look at the impact some questions can have on the client. For instance, let's say that a client has stated the following:

> Client: I felt terrible after Peter said that to me.
> Practitioner 1: Why do you feel terrible about that?
> Practitioner 2: It did sound awful, how else did it affect you?

Discussion points: In a small group (no more than six students) spend 10–15 minutes discussing each practitioner's response to the statement. Which question would you prefer and why? Write down some notes on these and compare these notes with those from other groups.

Most of us know what it is like to feel 'terrible'. However, it may be a slightly different experience for each individual. The question by Practitioner 1 is asking the client to give a rationale/reason why they felt the way they did. In other words it could be inferred by the client that the practitioner is making a judgement in which there is a right or a wrong answer. Generally speaking, questions that begin with 'Why' are usually very deep and require much thought on the part of the client. However, the question asked by Practitioner 2 is a much softer question; it reflects the client's feeling and it allows the client to expand on their earlier statement. This not to say that asking questions that begin with 'Why' is wrong. Rather, asking other softer questions might be a better option and they might elicit much more self-disclosure in the therapeutic relationship.

(f) Silence in the therapeutic relationship

When practitioners begin the skill of face to face communicating with clients about life's difficulties, moments of silence can seem like hours. However, a period of silence can have many meanings in the therapeutic relationship. More often than not, a period of silence allows the client and the practitioner to think and reflect quietly on what has been said previously. Both parties may be waiting for the other to take the lead again. Deciding who is to take the lead is usually made on the basis of what was last said in the interaction. It could be that the earlier part of the conversation has now finished and it is time to explore the topic from a different angle. In contrast, periods of silence could indicate that either the client or the practitioner is afraid of moving to a much deeper level in the topic. On the other hand, the client can use silence to frustrate the practitioner. While this may seem like a very negative view of some clients, on occasion some clients can challenge practitioners (Corey, 2005) or they may just choose to say nothing in response to questions (Hargie and Dickson, 2004). On such occasions the use of silence may indicate a hidden meaning and as such it must be acknowledged. If necessary its meaning should be explored by the client and the practitioner. However, silence should never at any time be looked upon as a threat to the therapeutic relationship. While it can be uncomfortable to practitioners in the early part of their career, it is a very useful component in the therapeutic relationship. As such both parties can use it to reflect on what has occurred and then move on with the topic.

An example of a caring response

Irrespective of whether the client has a history of self-harm with no suicidal intention or whether (s)he currently feels suicidal, the best caring response will incorporate a non-judgemental approach and active listening skills. Most, if not all, practitioners will already have some training in verbal and non-verbal communication skills. These skills are the same as those used in the major counselling/psychotherapy models. I must point out that their use here is an example of a caring response that demonstrates mental health first aid to a client who is in deep despair or in crisis. Readers may wish to follow up on these skills by referring to the Mental Health First Aid Program (Kitchener and Jorm, 2002), the ASIST programme (LivingWorks, 2004), or brief Crisis Intervention (Catalan *et al.*, 1984a, 1984b; Hawton and Catalan, 1987; Aguilera, 1994). All of these are very useful.

Case vignette 24

Peter was a 44-year-old man. He was married to Marge and they had three teenage children, two boys and a girl. Peter was previously employed in a local clothing business. He made his way up through all the different positions and had through his endeavours become sales manager with a small team. However, just over 14 months before his admission to hospital the business had to close down in face of stiff competition from larger and more competitive companies. The company started to accrue debts and employees were eventually made redundant. Peter received a redundancy package, which ensured that his family were looked after during his unemployment period. However, in the following months, Peter tried for a number of jobs but found that he was considered either too old or too well qualified. He has been unemployed since being made redundant.

In the last two months, Peter had become somewhat withdrawn, he had low self-esteem and he felt that he was a burden to everybody. The family were putting pressure on him to find a job and debts were beginning to mount. In the face of this additional pressure, he became very depressed and he went to see his GP. Peter did not admit to any thoughts of suicide but his GP was concerned. After consulting with both Peter and Marge, it was agreed that Peter be voluntarily admitted for assessment to the acute admission ward in the local mental health hospital. During the last four days in the ward his wife and children visited Peter on a regular basis. On the fifth day after a visit you notice that Peter is sitting alone at his bedside, he is frowning and seems somewhat preoccupied. How do you respond? *The words in italics are general comments on most such interactions.*

It must always be remembered that the big fear is that of suicide. In this brief caring intervention, the main goal will be to keep Peter safe and prevent suicide. When a client is actively attempting suicide, practitioners should not get physically involved but should immediately call for help. Any damage to the interpersonal relationship between the client and the practitioner will need to be repaired as soon as possible after any physical intervention. However, if a client is not actually attempting suicide, you do not need to call for assistance. The following approach to Peter's situation contains aspects of mental health first aid and brief crisis intervention therapy and may be quite helpful.

You: Hi Peter, I see that your wife and children have gone home. How did your visit go? *In the first instance, stay with Peter and ensure that he is not alone. This should not be forced and it may feel as if you are intruding but you are making a statement of wanting to be there with and for Peter. Sometimes just being there for the person is a very caring response* (Egan, 2006).

Peter: It went OK but it is a real bummer being in here. *Subtle statement about not wanting to be in hospital.*

You: Yes, I'm sure it is upsetting for you. I couldn't help noticing but you do look sad and I was wondering if that was anything to do with you being in here? *This demonstrates some empathic understanding and reflection of feeling. It also includes a very soft question that invites Peter to say more.*

Peter: Well I don't really want to be in here but I have tried everything else and it hasn't worked. Nobody wants to employ me, the funds are running out, I have started to go into debt and my family are pushing me to get back to work. I just don't know what to do about it. *Peter is suggesting that his unemployment is creating difficulties and his family are putting pressure on him.*

You: So you are upset because of the unemployment and debt situation and you feel that your family are putting you under pressure to get a job. *This paraphrases Peter's concerns and does not convey any judgement.*

Peter: That's right. It really is a mess, I feel useless and I have let my family down. Sometimes I think that life is not worth it. *Peter has now catastrophized the negative events in his life. He also gives a clue that he may have considered suicide. This statement MUST NOT be ignored.*

You: Yes, it does sound very serious Peter. Have you ever thought about killing yourself? *Here you acknowledge the seriousness of Peter's financial situation. Also, by directly asking about the possibility of suicide, you are indicating to Peter that you are not afraid to talk about it. This is not the time or place to make stupid statements such as 'Pull yourself together' or 'Things will work out' or 'Sure other people are worse off than you.' These statements are at best, less than useless and at worst they are judgemental in that you are minimizing the seriousness of his concerns.*

Peter: . . . *a brief silence ensues.* Well, things are pretty bad and I don't see any way out. I can't go to the bank because I have no income, I am so ashamed of what happened and so unable to do anything about it. It's really terrible and things have just got more and more on top of me. So in the last few weeks I have thought about suicide. It seems the best way out for all concerned. That is why I agreed to come in here but I told nobody about that. *The initial short silence indicates that Peter is thinking about what to say. Peter has said quite a lot here and it would be best practice to let him say what he wants to say without interruption. Your only response here should include good eye contact, a few head nods and maybe a few Hmm, Hmm. Only when Peter has finished would you consider a response.*

You: It seems to me that the main reason why you want to kill yourself is to do with all the negative events that have happened to you in the last 14 months. Are there any other reasons why you want to kill yourself? *You show good paraphrasing here. There is a temptation to repeat everything that Peter has said, but you have opted to acknowledge his reasons without any judgement whatsoever. In addition, you have given him the opening to mention other reasons for dying. It is best to explore all of the reasons for dying. At this time do not try to explore, contradict, or seek solutions to any of them. Just listen and let Peter disclose all his reasons.*

Peter: Well, my family think that I am a failure and at times I think that my friends do to. It is really embarrassing for me and I can't hold my head up in the neighbourhood. If things go on the way they are I think that we will have to sell our home to pay off our debt. So you can see where all this pressure is coming from. *Peter has stated additional reasons for dying. You will immediately note that one of his reasons for dying can also be a reason for living – he thinks his family think him a failure. This might be a blind spot and could be a trump card. There are other blind spots in the above statement as well (can you spot them?). For now we will focus on the family one. However, now is not the time to deal this possible trump card.*

You: So you think that your family and friends may think that you are a failure in life and that all this makes you feel the way you do? *You are now confirming Peter's reasons for dying.*

Peter: Yes, that's right . . . *Brief silence* . . . That's what I think.

You: Do you have any other reasons for wanting to kill yourself? *You are allowing him to ventilate any other possible reasons for dying.*

Peter: No, that's about it. I suppose things would be OK if I could get a job but they're not OK. *In the middle part of this statement, Peter has suggested a glimmer of hope that he wants to live. As he has not admitted any other reasons for dying, it is now time to move on.*

You: In what way did you plan to kill yourself? *A direct question that shows you are accepting what he says and that you are non-judgemental. Also, it maintains his focus on his death wishes and invites him to disclose his suicide plan.*

Peter: Well I haven't been taking the tablets the doctor prescribed and I have saved them up. I have heard that 20 tablets would be enough to kill me. It's my 45th birthday next week and I thought that I would have enough then and do it shortly after that. I don't like the idea of hanging myself, it seems too messy. *Here he has confirmed his suicide plan of how he is going to kill himself and when he is going to do it. You also know that he has a stash of tablets somewhere. In addition, you are very confident that he is not going to kill himself this night. Nonetheless, you will need to act on this information in a way that is within your Code of Conduct and that is acceptable to Peter.*

You: So you have saved up your medications and you want to take an overdose at some point after your birthday. *You are confirming his suicide plan.*

Peter: Yeah, that's right. All my problems will end then. *This part of the topic has now ended: you know his reasons for dying and you know his suicide plan. Also, you have demonstrated to Peter that you are genuine, non-judgemental and empathic. Now is a good time to up the ante and move Peter's thinking onto a new plane. For some time you have given Peter adequate time to reflect on his death orientation. Now is the time to move him over to a life-orientated focus by creating ambivalence in his thinking. (See Chapter 3 for more detail on ambivalence).*

You: Peter, you have told me all about your reasons for killing yourself but I also get the feeling that part of you wants to live. Can you think of any reasons for living? *Peter has for some time focused only on his death wishes. If you are to get him to want to live, you must first get him to think about reasons for living. Some authors have reported that clients who have attempted suicide have fewer reasons for living (Pinto, Whisman and Conwell, 1998). Also, because of the information in his case history (Case vignette 24) and in his story as told above, you are very much aware of a number of very positive blind spots (Luft and Ingham, 1963; Egan, 2006). Do not be tempted to list them here. Rather, try to get him to think of some. Remember that finding one good reason for living may be enough to keep him alive.*

Peter: . . . *brief silence* . . . Well not really. I have been so focused on my reasons for dying that I can't see any reasons for living. *The brief silence at the beginning has demonstrated that he has thought about it. He has opted to confirm his thoughts of suicide. Also, he uses the words 'I can't see any reasons . . .' This could be interpreted as meaning 'I don't want to see any reasons.' Now is a good time to pull the rug from under his suicide plan gently but firmly and to challenge at least one of his blind spots by playing one of the trump cards.*

You: Peter, what about your children? Are they not a good enough reason for living? *This is your biggest trump card and it will challenge his reasons for dying. It will also get him to focus on at least one reason for living.*

Peter: I don't think so. They think that I am a failure and before long they will know that I am a failure when we lose our home. *He is very much keeping to his suicide plan but he has now confirmed his fear that his children think that he is a failure.*

You: So you believe that your children think you're a failure? What will they think about you after you have killed yourself? *You have acknowledged his thinking but by asking him to focus on something he has not considered you have made him now look at life beyond his suicide. His wife is another blind spot and you have deliberately kept her out of the conversation at this stage. If needed, her part in opening up his blind spots can be explored at a later time. But not at this moment.*

Peter: . . . (*Brief silence*) . . . I didn't think too much about that. I just assumed the worst. I don't know what they think. Maybe, I need to think about things again. Oh, I don't know what to do. This is so painful and I am so confused. *This may sound like you have upset Peter. Well, in a way you have. For instance, he gave you, in his opinion, the best reasons to kill himself and you have just ruined his suicide plan. What has happened here is that you have created ambivalence in Peter. He has now moved onto safer ground. At this moment he does not know whether he wants to live or die. He needs to reconsider his options.*

You: A few times you have said that you are confused about what you want and I still get the feeling that a part of you wants to live. What are you thinking about now? *Here you have paraphrased what Peter has said and reflected his feelings. Also, you have given him an opening to say what he thinks now. This is giving him control again and it is also about you finding out the degree of risk there is now.*

Peter: . . . *brief silence* . . . Yes, I do feel really confused now. I was so set on killing myself that I didn't think of other important things. I thought that by killing me it would ease my pain and my family could get on with their lives. Now I am not so sure. *Peter is now ambivalent about his situation. However, he has moved slightly more towards the centre of a safe area and his risk of suicide has decreased. However, he is not over on the life side yet and he still has a stash of tablets hidden away somewhere. Now would be a good time to talk about how to keep him safe and for how long.*

You: It sounds to me that you have changed you mind about killing yourself? What do you think we should do to keep you safe and help you to work through the difficulties you are facing? *You have acknowledged and reinforced his change of mind. However, you have now very gently introduced the idea of partnership between you and him. Also you brought his safety into sharp focus and you have also asked him to focus on how to handle the future. This may seem like quite a shopping list for a short period of time but it does help to move him more into a life-orientated focus.*

Peter: Yeah, since I came in here you are the first person to really talk to me. I feel that it has helped me clarify some things and maybe, I need to talk more about what I need to do. What would you think? *Here he has acknowledged your help and he has brought you into the relationship. Also, he has affirmed for you that his risk of suicide is low and as a bonus that he is open to follow up therapy (if needed). He has also invited you to help decide what he needs to do next. This is a very positive statement from him.*

You: I'm glad that you think that this talk was helpful and of course you can talk to me at any time. However, it might be more helpful if you talked to one of our counsellors about your options. What would you think if I brought this up at the team meeting tomorrow and try to arrange an appointment for you with one of the counsellors? *You have acknowledged his positive comments about your help and asked him to consider therapy from a specialist practitioner. This offers him some hope for the future as well.*

Peter: Yeah, that might be helpful. At least then I can bounce my ideas and feelings about. Sometimes when I talk to my wife, we both get so frustrated. Maybe, it is time that I talked to a professional. *He has moved even further into the safe area and is on the life-orientated focus. Now would be a good time to go after the stash of medications and possibly make a no-suicide contract. The usefulness of a no suicide contract, or a no-self-harm contract is debatable. There are arguments for and against. Also, there is some evidence that they can be used in a punitive manner. I am not advocating that they must be used in all cases. I would argue that if it is needed, then it is one that is agreed by both parties and not forced on the client or for them to act on alone. It is an agreement by both parties in which both parties have to fulfil the objectives each has agreed to.*

You: I am really glad that you are no longer considering suicide. Also, at the team meeting tomorrow we can review whether or not you need the medications that you have been prescribed. But in the meantime, I am really concerned about the tablets that you have stashed away and as part of keeping you safe I would appreciate if you gave those to me now. Will you? *You have reinforced his current thinking and help him take another step in the direction of the safe side. He is gradually moving towards a life-orientated position. However, you realize that he is not entirely over there yet and in order to keep him safe you need to remove the means by which he has planned to kill himself.*

Peter: OK, I would appreciate if you didn't tell my wife about this. I would be really embarrassed and hurt if she found out. *Peter is making a request that may be difficult to keep. However, bearing in mind that most suicides and self-harm acts are carried out in secrecy or when the person is alone and nobody else knows about it, then it would not be right to agree to such a request. Again, it would be much more useful to get Peter to agree to his wife being informed but at a suitable time and with his consent.*

You: Well, I can't agree to that at this moment but I won't say anything to her without your consent. There might be advantages to letting her know about what has really happened, as sometimes it is best not to keep secrets. However, whether you should tell your wife is something that you can definitely discuss in therapy with the counsellor. What do you think? *You have not promised him false hope about this. However, you have suggested to him that telling his wife might be important and that he could discuss this point in therapy. This in effect gives him some degree of involvement in decision making.*

Peter: OK, I will agree to that as long as I know what is happening and what has been said to my family. *Peter now accepts the plan of action.*

You: Good, I am glad that you agree. Now let's go over what both of us have agreed to and then we will go and get that stash of tablets. *At this point you should review all of the agreed issues. This would include Peter affirming that he is no longer considering suicide. You will need to keep to your commitments, otherwise Peter will assume that you are full of false promises. If you cannot keep your (reasonably achievable) commitments, then why should he keep his? Peter now feels safe and you know that he is now safe. However, you both know that he needs additional therapy to consider his options. If you follow up on your commitments, then he will regain faith that others care for him and this might be the spur for him to refocus on what he needs to do to achieve employment in the future.*

At this point many clients feel a lot better as a direct result of someone taking a genuine interest in them; spending time with them and listening to them speak their mind. In many cases this is enough and client's go home and do well for the rest of their lives. Unfortunately, it does not always end that way and in statutory establishments such as hospitals or Community Mental Health Teams, practitioners need to feel very sure that all issues have been addressed before discharging a client. It can be more difficult for those practitioners who are self-employed and where clients just don't turn up after one session. These practitioners will not know whether the client has dealt with his/her difficulties or just did not want to come back into therapy. Nonetheless, much will depend on how the last interaction went and what action was agreed in therapy. In Peter's case above, he has agreed to certain action and this can quite easily be followed up.

If a client is considering suicide and lives alone, then this is a high-risk factor and could seriously complicate matters. As before, you need to ensure that the client is kept safe until (s)he can avail him or herself of other necessary therapy. For instance, after you have moved the client away from the death-orientated focus to the life side, it would be best that you get them to have a family member or friend stay overnight. Also, make sure that they agree not to take alcohol or drugs. Drinking alcohol can increase feelings of depression and loneliness. In addition, if the client has stockpiled medications, is going to use a gun, or a rope, the method must be removed for safe-keeping. It is much preferable if the client hands these over as it shows commitment towards keeping them safe. As with Peter, you will need to ensure that any no-suicide contract must also contain psychological interventions, if needed, to address the client's underlying emotional difficulties.

It is well known that those who repetitively self-harm are at very high risk of eventual suicide. However, self-harm is very much to do with the person coping with a stressor in their life rather than trying to end their life. For instance, Smith (1998) points out that self-harm is about control, where the person can control what they are doing and with that they have some control over their lives. Also, according to the Mental Health Foundation/Camelot Foundation (MHF/CF, 2006), young people who self-harm often feel that they can deal much more easily with physical pain than they can with emotional pain. To prevent clients from self-harming would therefore deprive them of this control and from using their chosen coping mechanism. Indeed, Pembroke (1998b) makes the case that depriving a client of their method of self-harm could result in much worse behaviour. She also suggests that making self-harm safer could be an option. However, this creates a major dilemma for health care authorities. For instance, custodial care regimes currently will not tolerate a client cutting themselves while in their care. This would breach their 'Maintain safety at all cost protocols'. It would also breach the codes of conduct for nurses and for other practitioners, because in these they are asked to maintain the clients' safety and ensure no harm. Currently there is a debate within nursing regarding nursing responses to self-harm and in particular when the client uses cutting. This debate includes issues around safer cutting. However, health care authorities will also need to review their stance and make recommendations as to how carers in their employment should respond to self-harm.

When I reflect back on Pat's story (Case vignette 1) I remember that the custodial care system did not work for him. In fact, it was very frustrating for him because we removed the only control he had in life. At that time, other staff and I did not understand what self-harm was about. Most of us associated it with suicide and therefore the main caring response was observation and ensuring no harm came to Pat. The cutting incident gave Pat and the staff something to focus on initially. However, it soon became clear that the behaviour was of secondary importance to Pat's feelings about himself and his life in general. In fact, his self-harm was a reflection of his inner feelings. When practitioners recognize and accept this, then maybe they will be able to respond in a more caring manner to clients who self-harm.

Nonetheless, in the case of self-harm, the intervention by a practitioner would, up to a point, have similarities to the intervention given to Peter. You cannot force an interaction but you can let the client know that you are interested in them and that you are there for them. Any intervention must employ all of the characteristics that have been previously mentioned including congruence, unconditional positive regard, and empathic understanding. This is very important as a great many of these clients will have had previous negative experiences from others including practitioners and they will, like anybody else, measure how trustworthy you are. If your verbal and your non-verbal language are congruent with each other, there is a fair chance that the client who self-harms will allow you to enter their world.

In any interaction where the client self-harms the focus of the interaction must be on the client and his/her feelings and not on their behaviour. This is because many people who self-harm dissociate themselves from the situation that is causing them despair. By focusing on the person behind the behaviour, exploring their experience and their feelings, and by helping them to understand what it is they are doing and why they are doing it, you will be trying to reconnect them with their own self. In so doing, you will demonstrate that someone does not judge them, but cares for them; is interested in them, and wants to hear what they have to say. In self-harm, short-term interventions may succeed in preventing self-harm for only a short while. A short-term fix is exactly that – a short-term fix; it is not a permanent solution. However, the root cause(s) of a client's anguish which is manifested in self-harm must, in the long term, be addressed through counselling/psychotherapy. Where any agreements are made between client and practitioner, they must be followed up. Not to do so may confirm the client's already negative perceptions of themselves and their situation and could possibly result in future suicide.

Summary

This chapter focused on caring responses to client's despair. There is ample evidence that custodial type practices have not worked and are still not working. These practices should be abandoned in favour of engaging with clients and helping them through their emotional despair. There is overwhelming evidence that engaging with clients: spending time with them, listening to their difficulties and allowing them to express their feelings, is what client's want. However, in order to help clients through personal difficulties, practitioners themselves need to become more aware of themselves and who they are. In demonstrating a caring attitude, practitioners need to display the following characteristics: (1) congruence, (2) unconditional positive regard and (3) empathic understanding. These characteristics are paramount in the therapeutic relationship (Rogers, 1961). If these are not present in the practitioner, then they will not be able to demonstrate a caring response and the therapeutic relationship will fail at the first hurdle.

While a caring response would include just being with the client (Egan, 2006), it also involves verbal engagement with the client. This is not counselling per se but is the ability of the practitioner to competently use their communication skills in a situation that requires mental health first aid. The object is to keep the client safe until they can avail of other more in-depth therapy. While being helpful in assisting a person through a crisis or feelings of despair, brief interventions do not solve the underlying emotional issues. Some of these issues may stem back to individual stressors but which now have become ingrained in the person's psyche. It is the negative narrative where the client believes the recurrent negative thoughts such as 'I am useless' or 'I never get anything right'. These issues, although allowing the person to be open to caring responses by genuine practitioners, will need to be addressed by other more in-depth therapy. Finally, the above example of a caring response is not just about demonstrating a set of verbal skills; there are also the non-verbal body language cues and other characteristics that are involved in the caring response. These are personal to all practitioners and, when combined, their presence will greatly assist them to develop the therapeutic relationship between themselves and their clients.

Therapeutic responses to suicide-related behaviour

8

In this chapter we will look at some synopses of therapeutic responses to suicide-related behaviour. In Chapter 7 an example of a short-term caring intervention was given. There is an acceptance among practitioners that many clients will benefit greatly from such a caring response but not all clients will find such benefits. First, there are individuals who focus so much on negative beliefs about themselves that at times it seems as if they are ingrained into their psyche. It is very difficult to remove such beliefs in a once off therapeutic encounter. Second, those individuals who repetitively self-harm are frequently in a (psychological/emotional) place where the only control they have in their lives is the degree of self-harm that they do to themselves. This is their way of coping with emotional despair. As mooted in Chapter 7, removing this coping mechanism without replacing it can transform the behaviour into something more dangerous. There has to be something in its place. This chapter focuses on those therapies that provide a more long-term response to suicide-related behaviour.

In Chapter 8 the following issues are explored:

1. A medical response – medications
2. A therapeutic response – additional notes
3. A therapeutic response – the assessment
   (a) Set induction
   (b) Assess events leading up to admission
   (c) Assess personal history
   (d) The care plan

4. A therapeutic response – problem management
5. A therapeutic response – challenging negative cognitions
    (a) The initial assessment
    (b) Making the A–C link
    (c) Making the B–C link
6. A caring and therapeutic response to self-harm

A medical response – medications

In this book the medical response has been selected for exploration at this point in order to deal with it and move on but not to dwell on it as the only solution to a client's psychological difficulties. There are neither anti-self-harm nor anti-suicide tablets. In addition, not everyone who shows evidence of suicide-related behaviour will be in a state of physiological anxiety. Some people can be quite calm and they are so because they have already made their decision as to how they are going to cope with issues that are creating despair in their lives. Some people can go to their deaths in a very calm way in the knowledge that tomorrow there will be complete peace in their lives. However, other people do present themselves to helping authorities while they are in a very high state of anxiety. In addition, they may already have survived what appears to be an attempted suicide. Conversely, their suicide-related behaviour may have been impulsive and they may have survived by chance rather than by planning.

Most people can relate to the feeling of anxiety. These feelings are those associated with their biological response to stress. If there is difficulty resolving the stressor then the person can experience distress and this can produce very unpleasant physical effects on the client. For instance, they may experience increased heart rate, increased blood pressure, increased respiration, headaches, sweatiness, nausea and feeling faint. These in turn can affect how they think. For example, they can create negative thoughts about themselves and these can cause them to become more worried and amplify the feelings of anxiety. Feelings of doom can develop and these can cause further worry and distress and can be amplified more. In brief, bio-psychological responses create a loop in which symptoms become more severe. The relief of such symptoms would be paramount in most people and therefore it would seem relevant that such relief should be obtained as soon as possible. However, the natural response would involve trying to find a solution to whatever is causing distress in the person. Then they would have to wait for the effects of the parasympathetic nervous system to come into effect in order to calm them. For some people, this process could take a lengthy period of time. In such cases a short course of anxiolytic medications may be prescribed to help calm the biological effects that the stressor creates within the client. Frequently the medication that is prescribed is one of the benzodiazepines. Unfortunately, these medications have had a long history of being very much abused and they can increase dependency (DHSS, 1984; Catalan and Gath, 1985). Things have not changed since then and these drugs, while being effective in controlling the biological effects of stressors, such as anxiety, do absolutely nothing about resolving the root cause of the stressor. They can and do produce a calming effect in a client who is anxious, distressed or even depressed. Because they do this the client may perceive the medication as a solution. Unfortunately, this would be a very false assumption.

All too often, drugs such as those from the anxiolytic group are prescribed to provide quick fixes and to help settle a client. They are effective in doing this and therefore have a very important function in terms of responding in times of crisis. However, it is emphasized here that they are not a long-term solution to stressors or life's difficulties. For instance, it has been suggested that anxiolytic medications should only be prescribed for short-term use in order to reduce the physical feelings of anxiety, calm the client and allow the client to access other therapies (DHSS, 1984). Thus, it has been well recognized for more than 20 years that these medications are not a solution in themselves but can be useful in helping a client get to the point where they can be helped to work towards the best possible solution to their stressor. The problem that a practitioner has is to decide when a client should stop taking the medication. It is at that point that they can communicate effectively and they can be helped to resolve or cope with those issues that are causing them despair. Where possible the anxiolytic medications should be done without and the client should be helped by other means to deal with events that elicit despair in them. This may seem like a very optimistic suggestion. Nonetheless, it has been reported that short-term crisis intervention techniques have been as equally effective as anxiolytic medications in the treatment of people in psychological distress (Catalan *et al.*, 1984a, 1984b) In addition, cognitive behavioural therapy has also been reported as being effective in the treatment of mild to moderate depression (Seymour and Groove, 2005).

However, clinical depression could be the main stressor in a client. The difficulty with this type of depression is that there are conflicting theories as to its origins. There are theoretical perspectives that suggest a purely biological reason for depression. As previously mentioned, these theories focus on the belief that low levels of serotonin or norepinephrine at the nerve synapses are the main cause of depression and also suicide-related behaviour. In this theoretical position it therefore follows that if the nerve synapse were able to recycle (reuptake) serotonin or norephinephrine then depression and also suicide-related behaviour would be reduced. However, while this may seem relatively straightforward and believable, it most certainly is not. Currently, the debate surrounding the links between low levels of serotonin or low levels of norepinephrine at the nerve synapses and the use of medications to correct this has been undermined by a number of issues. First, the levels of serotonin at the nerve synapses cannot be directly measured through normal screening. In fact, levels of serotonin are suggested by its waste metabolite 5-HIAA and these are found by examining cerebro-spinal fluid. This type of testing is not routine and may remain so for the foreseeable future. Second, antidepressant medication takes about three weeks to take effect and other factors such as environmental, situational and psychological may impinge on the client's emotional and mental well-being during that period. Third, Lynch (2005) challenged the medical profession to prove the biological basis of depression and the only answer suggested to him was that it was a working hypothesis rather than a concrete fact. Fourth, the report by Meek (2004) in the Consumers Association (Great Britain) suggests that antidepressant medications may be less than useless on some occasions. Fifth, there is increasing evidence that our diets can influence our emotional status. Currently, the type of food we eat, how it is processed, and what is in our food is under scrutiny. Sixth, there is evidence from the US Food and Drug Administration which suggests that some antidepressants have been implicated in increased suicide ideation in some clients (FDA, 2004, 2005).

However, it would also be unreasonable to portray antidepressant medication as being of no use on all occasions. For instance, Shea (2002, pp. 62–63) gives a case example of Pat who tries to do without her medication but finds that, without any additional stress in her life or any changes to her psychotherapy programme, she becomes suicidal again. Even though this example is somewhat anecdotal, it helps to remind practitioners that to discard the theories about the usefulness of medication might just be throwing out the baby with the bathwater. Nonetheless, there are inconclusive results about the effectiveness of medications in the treatment of suicide-related behaviour and what is needed is research into the usefulness of medications that is totally unbiased and that is totally independent of any influence by drug companies. At this moment it is highly unlikely that a medical approach alone will provide solutions for suicide-related behaviour in people.

When considering whether medications should be used in any specific case it is recognized here that the domain of prescribing medication is primarily a medical decision. However, it is also acknowledged that nurses are currently being trained in this skill as well. The argument whether medications should be prescribed in all cases of depression is debatable. It would very much depend on several issues such as: (1) how the assessment of the client's emotional or psychological needs is carried out, (2) what the issues are that the client feels are causing distress or despair in them, and (3) what the client has identified as the best possible care strategy for resolving their difficulties. Medications have their uses. However, whether they should be used in the treatment of needs to be carefully balanced in terms of the client's psychological needs. In responding to suicide-related behaviour they should not be the first line of treatment. However, they should be considered when the client has been made fully aware of the effects and the side-effects of the medication and of alternative therapies.

A therapeutic response – additional notes

As stated previously, in providing therapeutic care for clients who exhibit suicide-related behaviour, the practitioner's most powerful tool is the therapeutic relationship (s)he has with the client. All forms of therapeutic interventions will only develop from this relationship. Where it does not exist, then therapy itself will be unsuccessful. As mentioned in Chapter 7, the core qualities of the therapeutic partnership must apply if a human-to-human connection is to be made between client and practitioner. In Figure 5.1, both helplessness and hopelessness are shown as key elements on the path to suicide-related behaviour (McLaughlin et al., 1996; Abramson et al., 1998; Barbe et al., 2004). When a person feels helpless about an event that causes distress in them, it can be interpreted as having no control over that issue. Having no control over a stressful event can be a basis for self-harm. Similarly, feeling hopelessness about the future can be interpreted as having no future and this type of negative thinking can lead to suicide-related behaviour. Therefore, practitioners and clients need to consider the type of therapy that would help clients regain control over events in their lives or regain hope for the future.

Once the practitioner has established his/her genuineness with the client the all-important work of regaining hope for the future can begin. While mental health first-aid techniques are very useful, more often than not the client's psychological care will involve one of the major counselling therapies. Which type of therapy would be the most appropriate is a difficult question to answer. More often than not there is no one therapy that will suit all cases. However, in the case of suicide-related behaviour (including both self-harm and attempted suicide) the qualities of the practitioner as portrayed by Rogers (1951, 1961) theory will have a large part to play in whatever type of therapy is offered.

A therapeutic response – the assessment

This is the first step on the journey of recovery for the client. Assessment is a cornerstone of the helping relationship and requires collaboration between the client and the practitioner. The importance of a thorough assessment cannot be underestimated and there is some anecdotal evidence that such an assessment can be quite therapeutic for clients. In addition, it is very important that good record-keeping is maintained for legal reasons. Unfortunately, only a synopsis of the assessment can be given here. However, for more in-depth information the practitioner is directed towards Shea (2002) as an influential authority in the assessment of suicide risk in clients. For by this, all of the information gathered will be made use of during the client's care or therapy. Therefore, practitioners should take time over the assessment so that the client's psychological and emotional needs are identified. Frequently, a psychiatrist carries out the assessment of those at risk of suicide. However, since the seminal work of Catalan *et al.* (1980a, 1980b) government have recommended that other practitioners after appropriate training should be used in the assessment of clients at risk of suicide (DHSS, 1984). A similar recommendation is made here. Practitioners should be trained in the assessment of suicide risk and this training should be assessed in both knowledge and practical competence.

Currently, there is no one tool that can competently assess suicide intent or suicide risk in clients. Practitioners would therefore need to be able to draw on a number of assessment tools. For instance, practitioners should be knowledgeable and competently skilled in using a 'psychosocial assessment' and where necessary incorporating various scales such as Suicide Ideation Scale (Beck, Kovacs and Weissman, 1979); the Suicide Intent Scale (Beck, Schuyler and Herman, 1974; Pierce, 1977) and the Hopelessness Scale (Beck *et al.*,1974) into the assessment. In addition to these, it may be necessary to assess the severity of the client's depression and the Beck Depression Inventory (Beck *et al.*,1979) would be recommended here. During the assessment the practitioner needs to balance their use of self in attending and making the human-to-human connection with ensuring that the assessment is properly carried out. There are two ways of carrying out an assessment:

1. The practitioner brings to the assessment their experience, a set of questionnaires that includes pages to be written into, boxes to be ticked, and numbers to be assigned. Their approach to the assessment is very structured and rigid. The assessment is very much like an interview.

2. The practitioner brings to the assessment their experience and a notebook with blank pages. Their approach is structured but is flexible to allow the client to expand on issues of concern. The practitioner is very much aware of the assessment schedule. The assessment is very much like a conversation.

Discussion points: In a small group of fellow students spend between 10 and 20 minutes discussing the advantages and disadvantages of (1) using a pre-arranged set of questionnaires or (2) a blank notebook in the assessment. Which would your group use? What implications would each method have on the assessment? It is important to realize that neither method is better than the other. What is important is to understand the impact each method would have on the assessment as a whole and then to take steps to minimize this impact or find a compromise between both methods.

(a) Set induction

Before the assessment begins, the practitioner needs to reflect on the skill of set-induction (Hargie and Dickson, 2004). Most clients will be very anxious about meeting a practitioner and having an assessment. Therefore it is very important that you put the client at ease. Remember that it is the client who makes the decision to attempt suicide or self-harm. Similarly, they will decide whether they will want to talk to you or to any other practitioner. It is well known that first impressions are lasting. For instance, the environment where the assessment will be held and how the practitioner (you) present yourself to the client will determine how far the relationship will develop. Besides your verbal and non-verbal signals, your presentation will also include your mode of dress and how welcoming the physical environment is. Greeting the client and shaking his/her hand might help them to relax. The offer of a cup of tea would be optional but also might be helpful. In order to physically tune into the client, you should make use of the components as outlined in the acronym SOLER (Egan, 2006). For instance, the seating could be arranged at a very slight angle to each other. Being too square may frighten the client. In the case of visually impaired clients, don't forget to aim your voice. During the initial friendly pleasantries, it would be very helpful if you gained permission from the client to do one of the following: (1) record the assessment using a tape or video recorder; (2) take written notes; or (3) have a second person take written notes. Each of these suggestions has limitations but each also has advantages. It would also help to let the client know that whatever notes are taken will be checked with them before the assessment ends. If a tape/video recording has been taken, the client should have access to a copy of the tape. Also, this would be the best time to talk to the client about the extent and the limits of confidentiality.

Discussion points: In a small group of fellow students spend between 10 and 20 minutes discussing the advantages and disadvantages of each of the three methods of recording details about the assessment. Which would your group use and why. Also, discuss the entire set induction as outlined above. What changes, if any, would you make and why? Compare your suggestions with students in another group.

Initially, it would be helpful if the client was encouraged to talk about him or herself in a very general way – things like where they live, who their family members are, and who their friends are. This will put the client at ease and also gather some very relevant details. For instance, you may find some of the client's (positive) blind spots located in information gathered here.

(b) Assess events leading up to admission

The practitioner (you) should gently move into an in-depth exploration of the events that have led up to the client's suicide-related behaviour. This is probably the most crucial part of the whole assessment. First, let the client tell you their story in the way they see fit. Sometimes, the story will be blurted out in a very confused manner. Remember that you are not in a hurry and the client must realize that they have time and more importantly – your attention. At other times, the story will unfold almost with a blow-by-blow account of who said what and who did what. At this stage your job will be to demonstrate empathy through your verbal skills (paraphrasing, reflection and questioning) and also through your non-verbal body language.

If the client has been admitted following suicide-related ideation, then the events leading up to it and future risk of suicide will need to be assessed. These can be carried out with help from the Scale for Suicide Ideation (Beck, Kovacs and Weissman, 1979) and the Hopelessness Scale (Beck *et al.*, 1974). If the client has been admitted following an attempted suicide or self-harm, then the events leading up to the admission and issues about the actual behaviour would need to be fully addressed. For instance, practitioners would be very interested to know what the person's intention was at the time of the behaviour. Using a triangulation process can check their intention. For instance, the client may self-disclose their intention during the telling of their story, the Suicide Intent Scale (Beck, Schuyler and Herman, 1974) can be woven into the assessment, and asking them directly – 'What was your intention at the time of the behaviour? ' This is probably the crux of the whole assessment. You do need to learn as much about the client's suicide plan as is possible and the more information you have about their plan the more likely you are to measure the extent of the person's intention to commit suicide in the future (Shea, 2002). In addition, by focusing on their suicide plan you are letting the client vent their death wishes and this demonstrates that you are interested in them and paying attention. There are a number of self-disclosures that would warrant considering a client at a serious risk of suicide in the future. These are:

1. They have recently suffered a serious loss (separation, divorce, bereavement or unemployment).
2. They have expressed very little hope for the future.
3. They have attempted suicide before or have a previous history of self-harm.

4. They have already made a suicide plan and have tried to keep it secret.

5. They have considered various suicide methods and have settled on one particular method.

6. They have planned when to carry out their suicide.

7. They have already made preparations (made a will, given away property etc.)

The client's intent during the assessment may be different to what it was at the time of the attempted suicide or self-harm. For instance, in Stephen's story (Case vignette 4), he scored very high on the Suicide Intent Scale (Beck, Schuyler and Herman, 1974) when it was measured against his attempted suicide behaviour. However, other aspects in his assessment made my mentor and myself come to the conclusion that he was now at a low risk of future suicide. For instance, he made it very clear on more than one occasion that he was glad to be alive and he was thinking of going back to his home town. In these snippets of information there was, in his case, a semblance of hope for the future. It seemed, in my opinion, that the assessment process had a therapeutic effect on Stephen. In contrast, in Elizabeth's story (Case vignette 5) she woke up from her ordeal and was so disappointed to see us and not meet St Peter. She was really angry and her use of profane language shocked her family. Her reaction suggested that she was, at that point, still at high risk of suicide. Subsequent discussions (evaluations) during the day found that she had mellowed in her temper but was still at high suicide risk. However, not all clients will present their intentions as clearly as Stephen or Elizabeth and practitioners would be unwise to leave this important part of the assessment without, in their professional judgement, a clear indication of the client's current risk of future suicide.

(c) Assess personal history

At this point you will explore the client's history from early childhood to current day. Some experts might say that this is superfluous and that it throws up too many red herrings. Maybe so, however, while many stressors are in the here and now, sometimes stressors come from negative experiences in one's past life. For instance, there are clues to future suicide and Shneidman (2005, p. 2) makes the point that 'childhood matters; parents count; bad luck is bad precisely because it tends to tar the future'. Therefore, it is useful to explore the client's development and experiences from childhood through to the present day. Opening questions such as 'How would you describe your childhood? ' and 'What memories of your childhood are most prominent? ' are quite useful. These sample questions allow clients to talk freely about their childhood and their school days. As before, let the client tell his/her story. Use active listening skills and be on the look out for blind spots in the story. In adolescence the questions would be similar but would include an exploration of the client's relationships within the family, with outside friends and the beginnings of sexual orientation. For instance, where did the client fit into their family: caretaker, hero, clown, lost child, or guru? The family is a very important entity for all persons, including the client. However, it is unfortunate to realize but important to acknowledge that the family can also be the setting for many of life's difficulties (Bradshaw, 1988, 1996). Also, who were their friends and where are these friends now? When did the client have their first sexual encounter? How did they get on in relationships? Depending on the age of the client, other issues that may require assessment could include work, marriage/living with a partner, how their own children (if any) are progressing, history of substance abuse, and any history of mental illness in the family. These latter issues will produce useful information about the client that can be used in future therapy. For instance, some of the client's (positive) blind spots could be located in this part of the assessment. As demonstrated in Chapter 7, being able to call upon these blind spots at the appropriate time could give the astute practitioner an edge and the client a very powerful reason for living.

On completion of the assessment you should check your notes with the client. Read over them and then summarize the main points. From these, both you and the client will identify:

1. the difficulties the client is facing;
2. the extent to which the client can exercise control over the difficulties (Barker, 2001);
3. what it is that the client wants to achieve;
4. what steps/objectives the client needs to take to achieve their aim.

(d) The care plan

When the client is not fully involved in the assessment and has not agreed to the care plan, then it will not work. Therefore, it is vitally important that there is collaboration between the client and the practitioner and that both agree a set of objectives that are needed to achieve the aim. Sometimes gaining the collaboration of the client can be quite difficult to achieve. However, if you have taken adequate steps in the 'set induction' and demonstrated at least an acceptance of the client (Rogers, 1951) then there is more than a good chance that collaboration will be achieved and the basis of the therapeutic relationship will be set. The care plan need not be set in stone but it is a guide along which the practitioner and the client can move along. For instance, it may become apparent at some point that achieving the initial aim would be unrealistic. In such cases it will need to be reviewed as to what is achievable. Nonetheless, an agreed step-by-step programme will need to be put in place. In this plan it will be specified what is to be done and by whom. Recently the Sainsbury Centre for Mental Health (2006), in a case vignette (Barry), reported that when Barry was assessed that he felt as if he were cut open. All his past was dug up and just left there. If the practitioner did something with it, it would have been OK but nothing was done with it, it was just left there. Barry was really upset with this. The point is made that assessments are not done for the point of providing information for the assessor and then doing nothing about it. Every scrap of information that has been gathered in the assessment must be put to use in follow-up therapy. Many practitioners think about how to predict future suicide in clients. One answer lies in how effectively the client's suicide risk is assessed. Shneidman (2005) makes the point that there are clues in a person's history that will predict future suicide. In assessing clients following suicide-related behaviour, skilled practitioners should be able to identify from their case history their potential for future suicide.

A therapeutic response – problem management

The case for moving from a medically orientated model of mental health care to a more person-centred model is well acknowledged (NICE, 2004b; SCMH, 2006). There are quite a number of very relevant counselling theories in use (Corey, 2005); however, there are few actual models. One such model is that described by Egan (2006). This model has two main goals and for reasons of clarity they are stated here:

1. to help clients manage their problems in living effectively and develop unused and missed opportunities more fully;
2. to help the client become better at helping themselves in their everyday lives.

While this model includes problem management, it also focuses on empowerment. Also, while the model is to some degree led by the practitioner, it is the client who has control over all decisions. In other words the client is involved in the process and heavily involved in the decisions. The model is best used for events in the client's recent past or events that are current and that create difficulties in the client's life. Thus, one can immediately detect that it would not be suitable for all cases where clients present with suicide-related behaviour. Nonetheless, when considering a client's current difficulties, the model has three stages and to demonstrate how these are applied I will give a synopsis of Mark's case history

(Case vignette 22). While Mark's case is given as an example of how the Egan's model worked in this instance, it is important to mention here that for Mark, as in many cases, the process did not follow in a logical step-by-step programme. There were difficulties along the way and on occasions sub-stages had to be revisited and ground had to be regained. For instance, in stage 1, his initial priority was to tell his employees first, rather than his parents. He worked through this decision for a time but then had to retrace his steps when he 'discovered' that he could manage his staff but his real difficulty was in telling his elderly parents. I am sure that many others could easily have told Mark that. However, that decision is not theirs to make. In this model, Mark has to work through his decisions until he knows that the one he has chosen is the right one for him.

(i) **Current scenario (What's going on?):** *This is stage 1 and it has three sub-stages. In brief, it is very much like an assessment stage but is focused more on the client's perspective. For instance, in this stage the client will tell their story without unnecessary interruption, blind spots will be sought and challenged and the client will decide what (s)he needs to do now.*

For instance, Mark allowed me to take notes and in his own words he told his story. He started off by talking about himself, his younger brothers and sisters and his elderly parents. At age 21 he started his own company and within four years it had become a success. He liked to lead from the front, be in control, be the front man, entertain his clients, and personally make the deals. Life was very busy but also very good for him. When he was caught drunk in charge of a vehicle, his thoughts focused on the shame it would bring to his parents and his younger siblings. Also, he knew that he would lose his driving licence and felt that this would cause his company to collapse. He felt guilty over his behaviour and shame that he had let down his family and staff. These were the reasons that he started to consider suicide-related behaviour. In challenging his blinds spots, he eventually acknowledged his own talents in building a small company and how successful he had become. He also acknowledged the love of his family and the number of friends he had. This helped in moving him from a death-orientated position to a life-orientated position and the possibility of hope in the future. At this point Mark was encouraged to think about what would be the most important thing for him to work on at that moment. He *eventually* decided that his family and his staff members were most important to him.

(ii) **Preferred scenario (What solutions make sense for me?):** *This is stage II and it also has three sub-stages. In these sub-stages the practitioner helps the client develop a sense of hope about the future. The client's imagination is encouraged so as to list all possible options. The client will then explore possible, even some unrealistic, choices that they have and craft these into ways that can help them change. The third sub-stage is about the client's commitment. What is it they are willing to 'pay' for what* *they want? This is essentially a search for incentives and frequently it will involve some personal change.*

In this stage Mark was asked to pose some potential solutions. This involved 'brainstorming tactics' and Mark was asked to write down his suggestions. Among his potential solutions were 'Talk to his staff', 'Talk to his parents', 'Talk to his brothers and sisters'. He was also encouraged to think of some imaginative solutions. He also suggested 'Run off to England', 'Go to the USA for a year or two'. *I have to admit that, in this stage, Mark made some very funny and also some unprintable suggestions.* No effort was made to contradict any suggestions, no matter how outrageous they were. This was about letting him be as realistic or unrealistic as possible. In the second sub-stage he reviewed how realistic each suggestion was. One particular question was very important here 'Of all your suggestions, which do think would be the most realistic?' The outcome of these discussions was that he chose as his main priority to 'Talk to his parents first'. *In Mark's case this decision did not come easily but it did come eventually.* In the next sub-stage Mark needed to review his commitment to achieving what he had now decided. In this part there is a price to pay and the price he had to consider was whether he could afford to 'lose face and be able to withstand the disappointment and possible anger from his elderly parents?' In rationalizing this sub-stage, Mark felt that the reaction from his parents would be immediate and short-term and that he would lose his licence for a year but could get it back in six months. However, he thought that his suicide would cause long-term difficulties for his whole family, his friends and his staff. He therefore came to the conclusion that talking to his parents would be the best way forward.

(iii) Action strategies (How do I get what I need or want?): *This is stage III in Egan's model. It also has three sub-stages. In this sub-stage the focus is on the activities the client needs to do so as to achieve what it is they want. In other words they are planning the potential activities. In general, the client will brainstorm various strategies, explore each for the best fit and then decide what it is they need to do first, second and so on.*

In the first sub-stage of stage III, we brainstormed various ways (strategies) of how he was going to tell his parents about his impending court case. Again Mark was asked to write these down and he made a number of suggestions. These included: 'Write them a letter', 'Tell a family member and then getting them to tell my parents', and 'Just tell them and get on with my life'. As before, none of his suggestions was contradicted and more were asked for. On completion of the activity, he was asked, 'Which of these do think will be the most likely to work? ' Mark went through the strengths and weaknesses and also factors or threats that might obstruct potential strategies. Eventually, he decided that the best strategy would somehow involve his gently talking to his parents and letting them know what had happened and what he intended to do. This was still Mark's big diffi-culty. He now accepted that he had to tell them. However, he did not know how he was going to tell them. In the final sub-stage of Egan's model (the plan) it was (*eventually*) agreed that Mark would: (1) perform some role-play exercises in which Mark would be himself and talk to me as if I were his parents and (2) tell his parents at an opportune moment after he had adequate practice and felt ready to do it.

Mark had several role-play sessions before he felt comfortable in arranging to talk to his parents. The role-play involved counteracting a number of potential threats such as setting up a meeting with only his elderly parents and that did not arouse their suspicion or cause them unnecessary worry. Nor should it arouse the suspicions of his siblings. It also had to include a place where they could talk in private. Additionally, role-play included what he was going to tell them and how he was going to say it. This sub-stage required much discussion and was at times fraught with hazards. Nonetheless, role-play proved effective and Mark agreed on the implementation of his plan after a somewhat hard won battle. While we agreed to follow-up in three months' time, I did not see Mark for almost a year. He telephoned for an appointment and he told me of his progress since our last meeting. He had told his parents and his family, he lost and regained his licence, his business was still flourishing and he no longer drank alcohol during business lunches. In addition, and as a bonus, he told me that he was able to use the learning experience he had in therapy to resolve a family row between two of his younger siblings and their elderly parents.

A therapeutic response – challenging negative cognitions

Ever since the battle for behaviourism (Watson and McDougall, 1929), both cog-nitive therapy and behaviour therapy have remained poles apart. However, from the 1970s both cognitive psychology and behavioural psychology have begun to recognize each other's central role in treating emotional and behavioural prob-lems in people. Currently, behaviour therapy tends to be combined with cognitive therapy and is called cognitive behavioural therapy (CBT). In brief, cognitive behaviour therapy is based on the reasoning that a client's behaviour and mood are determined by the way they structure their world (Beck *et al.*,1979). In other words there is a relationship between life events, the way a client thinks and how they behave and express their emotions. From a CBT perspective a client's difficul-ties stem from cognitive distortions (negative thoughts) about the self, which are learned and are self-defeating (Russell and Morrill, 1989). This is very relevant in suicide-related behaviour where many clients will have very negative thinking patterns about themselves. For example, some people make very dysfunctional assumptions about themselves, which, at some point, they begin to believe. These assumptions, once activated, can produce an upsurge of negative automatic thoughts about the self (Mahoney, 1974; Fennell, 1989; Moorley, 1995; Sheldon, 1995). These thoughts can be quite distressing for the client because they occur spontaneously and they are always very pessimistic about all or any aspects of the client's past, present or future life. The interruption of this circle of negative automatic thoughts is crucial if a person is to return to a more stable emotional and psychological state. In order to address this, these negative thoughts are challenged and cognitive restructuring is used to change maladaptive beliefs (Mahoney, 1974; Meichenbaum, 1977; Moorley, 1995; Deffenbacher, 1996; Lam, 1997; Maris, Berman and Silverman, 2000).

Cognitive behaviour therapy is a structured time-limited problem-solving approach that aims to modify faulty information processing that characterizes depression. It has been shown to be useful treatment for depressed or suicidal persons (Beck *et al.*, 1979; Free, Oei and Sanders, 1991; Atha, Salkovskis and Storer, 1992; Barker, 1992; Moorley, 1995; Sheldon, 1995; Dobson and Jackman-Cram, 1996; Lam, 1997; Maris, Berman and Silverman, 2000; Shea, 2002). It uses behaviour modification techniques but also incorporates cognitive restructuring to change maladaptive beliefs (Mahoney, 1974; Meichenbaum, 1977; Moorley, 1995; Deffenbacher, 1996; Lam, 1997; Maris, Berman and Silverman, 2000). Cognitive restructuring provides a selection of options in problem-solving situations, increases coping abilities, and allows clients to assume control over symptom management (Blair, 1996). However, it pays little attention to childhood memories other than to clarify current difficulties and the practitioner actively cooperates with the client in exploring experiences, setting up activity schedules, and arranging homework assignments (Beck *et al.*, 1979).

In implementing cognitive behaviour therapy, practitioners use the ABC model (Trower, Casey and Dryden, 1989). The 'A' is known as the activating event (or stressor), 'B' is the client's belief or interpretation of this event, and 'C' is the person's behavioural or emotional response. This is represented in Figure 8.1.

What is noticeable in this model is that the activating event (A) leads to a client interpreting the event and formulating beliefs about it (B). Also, one can see that it is the client's beliefs (B) about the event that causes the consequences (C). However, what is very clear is that the activating event (A) does not cause the consequences (C). Therefore, the model pivots on the client's belief systems (B). These belief systems form the basis of the client's cognitive distortions. Some of these cognitive distortions can be so ingrained in the person's psyche that they are really very difficult to change. Nonetheless, in many cases cognitive distortions are amenable to cognitive restructuring. Also, while Rudd, Joiner and Rajab (2001) make the point that cognitive restructuring is but one component in the

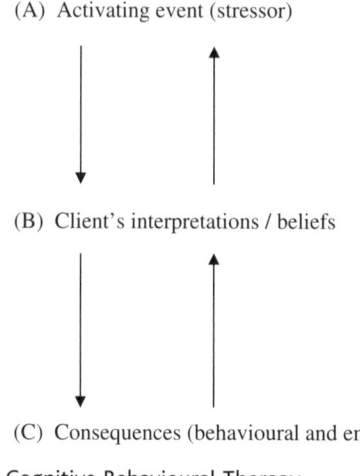

(A) Activating event (stressor)

(B) Client's interpretations / beliefs

(C) Consequences (behavioural and emotional)

Fig. 8.1 The ABC of Cognitive Behavioural Therapy.

treatment of suicide-related behaviour, they also state that it has a central role. Let's look at a synopsis of a case study to help clarify matters.

Case vignette 25

Maurice is a 37-year-old divorcee with two teenage children from his previous marriage. It took him a long time to recover from his divorce but he gradually built himself up and eventually moved on. A close friend introduced him to Jenna and they went out on a blind date. They got on very well and began dating in a steady relationship. Maurice was very worried that he might not be able to satisfy her sexually as it had been a while since he had been with a new partner. Their first attempt at sexual intercourse was a let-down for both. Nonetheless, Jenna was kind and very patient and both of them worked at it. Eventually their sex life began to thrive. Unfortunately, after 7 months, Jenna ended the relationship for no particular reason. Maurice blamed himself for the break-up. He saw this as his last chance at building a relationship. He felt that it was to do with his lack of sexual prowess and felt that he was on the verge of becoming impotent. He became depressed, began to isolate himself and began to think that Jenna was talking about him behind his back. Eventually he went to his GP who prescribed a course of antidepressants for him. He went home, opened a bottle of vodka and took the tablets. However, he telephoned the Samaritans to talk to them about what he had done. When he collapsed they contacted the emergency services and he was found in a comatose state. He was taken to the accident and emergency department and after having his stomach contents washed out he was transferred to the medical ward. After he was seen and assessed by a mental health liaison nurse he was referred for counselling.

(a) The initial assessment

As previously stated the practitioner must exhibit the core skills of acceptance, genuineness and empathy. In addition, the skills used in set induction also need to be employed. Initially, the practitioner used active listening skills and let Maurice tell his story. In telling his story Maurice was very anxious and his depression was very pronounced. On completion of his story the practitioner and Maurice talked about what cognitive behaviour therapy (CBT) entailed. The practitioner produced a blank piece of paper and he wrote down the letters A, B and C and he used these to illustrate Figure 8.1 above and inform Maurice what CBT was about. Also, they discussed Maurice's expectations from therapy. Although Maurice still had suicidal thoughts, he indicated some hope for the future, by saying, 'I would like to move on with my life.' *At this stage the practitioner will have got an overview of Maurice's difficulties and both Maurice and the practitioner will also have made some judgement about whether CBT would be the best form of therapy for him. In general, the main assessment and the basis for CBT would involve the following five steps:*

1. Assess the A component.
2. Assess the C component.
3. Link the A component to the C component.
4. Assess the B component.
5. Link the B component to the C component.

Some practitioners might suggest assessing the C component first and then the A component. Others will assess A before C. However, what is important is that A and C components are best assessed before the B component (Trower, Casey and Dryden, 1989).

(b) Making the A–C link

In this brief synopsis we will focus on the link between the A and the C components and then we will move on to linking the B component with the C component.

> Practitioner: It seems that your attempted suicide was a result of things that were going on in your life. Of all the difficulties that you mentioned, which would you want to talk about first?
> Maurice: I suppose I find it really hard to go out and meet other people.
> Practitioner: OK, how did you feel the last time you went for a night out?

Maurice: It was very strange at first. I went to a pub that Jenna and I used to go to but I didn't know anybody and then I felt very lonely. Imagine being lonely in a pub. I just didn't have the courage to go and talk to someone. Then a few of Jenna's friends came in and looked in my direction. I felt like I was going to collapse so I left in a hurry.

Practitioner: So, what you are saying is that you had difficulty enough going out in the first place but when Jenna's friends looked at you, you felt as if you were going to collapse.

Maurice: Yeah, that's about right.

Practitioner: OK, I'll write down 'Jenna's friends looked at me' in column A and I will write down 'I felt like I was going to collapse' in Column C. Is that OK with you?

Maurice: Yeah that's OK.

This interaction has been cut short at this point as the main point here was to demonstrate to Maurice that he had made a link between the A component (Jenna's friends looked at him) and the C component (felt as if he were going to collapse). In other words he was blaming an event for the way he felt.

(c) Making the B–C link

Practitioner: What thoughts were going through your mind when you noticed that Jenna's friends were looking at you?

Maurice: I thought that Jenna had said something to them and that they were talking about me.

Practitioner: I'll write this down in the B column 'I thought that Jenna's friends were talking about me.' What sort of things do you think that they were saying?

Maurice: . . . *brief silence.* . . . Well, Jenna knows a lot of things about me; some are good and some are not so good. And you know what women are like; they always talk to each other about men and such. So I thought that Jenna talked about me and said some nasty things about me.

Practitioner: Right, I will write that down in column B as well. OK, let's look at what we have got here. *Both looked at what was written on the paper (Figure 8.2) and the practitioner pointed out that the B component (Maurice's beliefs) comes between the A component and the C component.*

Practitioner: What do you think caused you to feel as if you were going to collapse? Was it Jenna's friends looking at you or the thoughts in your head?

Maurice: I suppose my own thoughts were a big part of it.

Practitioner: In what way were your thoughts a big part?

Maurice: ... *brief silence* ... I think that she (Jenna) might have said to them that I was useless in bed or something like that and that's what I think that they were talking about.

Practitioner: So, what you're saying is that you thought that Jenna was talking to her friends about your sex life and that they were talking about you among themselves. *The practitioner is trying to confirm the B–C link.*

Maurice: Yeah, that's what I thought.

Practitioner: OK, what evidence do you have that they were talking about your sex life? *This is an early attempt to undermine Maurice's cognitive distortion.*

Maurice: I don't have any evidence because I couldn't hear what they said; I just assumed that that was what they were talking about. *Maurice is beginning to question his belief about Jenna's friends talking about him.*

The above example is a very much abridged version and Figure 8.2 serves to give a visual representation of how the cognitive distortion (negative beliefs) can lead to the emotional and behavioural consequences. The above example also briefly demonstrates the basic principles of challenging a client's negative beliefs about themselves. The process of cognitive reconstruction would consist of the client finding evidence that his negative beliefs about himself were false. Therapy would take place over a period of time and the number of sessions would depend very much on the client's needs. Nonetheless, therapy could include: (1) socratic dialogue with the practitioner to undermine negative beliefs and find hidden

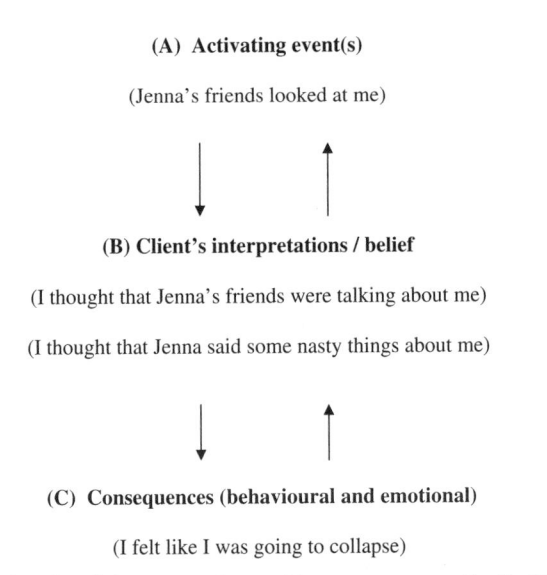

(A) Activating event(s)

(Jenna's friends looked at me)

(B) Client's interpretations / belief

(I thought that Jenna's friends were talking about me)

(I thought that Jenna said some nasty things about me)

(C) Consequences (behavioural and emotional)

(I felt like I was going to collapse)

Fig. 8.2 Linking the client's interpretations with consequences: the B–C link.

strengths; (2) role-playing in preparation for stressful events; and (3) homework that has been agreed between client and practitioner. In brief, cognitive reconstruction would occur as a result of the client confronting negative beliefs about him or herself with contradictory evidence that they have collected and appraised (Corey, 2005). For instance, even though it was Jenna who broke up with Maurice, while in Socratic dialogue with the practitioner, he came to the conclusion that she did not harbour any ill will against him. Therefore, one part of Maurice's homework was to return to the same pub and if any of Jenna's friends were to come in, he was to go and say hello to them. After role-playing the scene, he did meet and say hello to them and he found that he got on well with them. This in turn eventually gave him the confidence to talk to other women. Another cognitive distortion in Maurice's case study was explored in a similar fashion. For example, his impotence was attached to his belief that he wouldn't be able to have an erection. The negative thought perpetuated the impotence but with the help of Socratic dialogue regarding his past sexual experiences and with specific homework instructions, Maurice found that his impotence was temporary and due to his own negative beliefs about himself. There was improvement in this area also.

A caring and therapeutic response to self-harm

Responding to self-harm can be quite difficult for practitioners. This is because they usually have very little, if any, training or education regarding the needs of people who self-harm. Indeed, quite a few authors have called for increased training in relation to communicating with and caring for those who self-harm (Whittington and McLaughlin, 2000; Buston, 2002; McAllister et al., 2002; Anderson, Standen and Noon, 2003; Crawford et al., 2003; Eastwick and Grant, 2004; Friedman et al., 2006; MFF/CF, 2006). Many of these calls refer to the lack of communication skills in practitioners; negative attitudes by practitioners towards those who self-harm; and lack of support and guidance for practitioners involved with those who self-harm. In addition, adolescents who self-harm expect to be judged harshly and told off for wasting time (Dorer et al., 1999). Also, they feel guilty and ashamed; have difficulty in talking about their self-harm and are afraid of the response they get (MHF/CF, 2006). In response to these concerns, adolescents who self-harm frequently talk to their peers rather than to professionals. There is no doubting the seriousness of the issues that need to be resolved if care for those who self-harm is to be improved by those in the caring professions.

Some of the difficulties that underlie self-harm are issues like relationship difficulties, loss (separation/parental divorce), abuse (physical, sexual, psychological), and bullying. In addition, Bradshaw (1988, 1996) makes the point that rules and systems within the family can create difficulties for all family members. However, the negative effect of poisonous pedagogy or the no-talk rule within the dysfunctional family system will more than likely create serious emotional and psychological difficulties for growing children. It is known that difficult issues within the family do result in self-harm (McLaughlin, Miller and Warwick, 1996; Dorer *et al.*,1999). Furthermore, while hopelessness about the future is correlated with attempted suicide and suicide, other authors (McLaughlin, Miller and Warwick, 1996) report that hopelessness is also linked to self-harm.

So now that we have reminded ourselves about some of the causal factors that underlie self-harm in a person, in what way can the caring services and practitioners respond? There are a number of potential responses that may help the client who is self-harming. First of all, managers and practitioners alike need to look at the type of service they are currently providing. There is evidence that when practitioners try to understand clients who self-harm and respond positively to their needs, then it can help clients improve their self-esteem and develop hope for the future (Lindgren *et al.*, 2004). Other authors suggest that being friendly and non-judgemental is beneficial (Dorer *et al.*, 1999; Burgess, Hawton and Loveday, 1998). In addition, McAllister and Estefan (2002, p. 580) report that a client felt that the following response from a nurse was very gentle:

> I am not going to pretend I understand why you did this, but I think you must have been in a lot of pain inside. I'm not sure what I can do to help, but I'll listen if you want to talk to someone. You look pretty uncomfortable, sort of like you might want to get out of here quickly, so you mightn't want to talk to me, and that's okay too. We can just chit chat or be silent. I'll just take my lead from you.

For whatever reason, there is a sense of distrust of health care practitioners by many of those who self-harm. This distrust is unfortunately targeted towards well-meaning and very professional practitioners as well. Therefore, the onus is on all practitioners who come into contact with those who self-harm to demonstrate their genuineness and their trustworthiness. The appreciation by the client of the above statement echoes Pembroke's (1998b) positive sentiments towards an accident and emergency nurse who treated her with respect. Although anecdotal, these suggest that a very human-to-human connection is probably a very important response in the initial stages. Sometimes just being with the client and spending time with them would be appreciated. Therefore, it would seem that practitioners, who exhibit the personal and professional qualities as discussed in Chapter 7, should find it much easier to engage with and communicate with those who self-harm.

Currently there is an ongoing debate about the possibility of safer self-harm. However, as stated earlier, within current statutory health care regulations, safer self-harm is not an option. Nonetheless, both professional bodies and health authorities will need to get to grips with it in terms of how practitioners should intervene. I am not of the opinion that simply handing out clean razor blades is a possible answer. It might well be part of the answer but it is not the whole answer. There must also be a human element to it as well. If it comes to pass that safer self-harm is endorsed by the statutory services and supported by professional bodies, will practitioners stay with clients and support them while they carry out their self-harming behaviour? This would be the ultimate demonstration of support and acceptance of the client by the practitioner. In her influential article Louise Pembroke (1998b) makes suggestions for safer self-harm. She also makes the point that practitioners should 'accept the client's need to self-harm as a valid method of survival, until survival is possible by another method' (Pembroke, 1998b, p. 24). In this latter statement she is suggesting that there are alternatives to self-harm but that clients need to be able to access them. Recently, it has been suggested that clients may be able to self-manage their self-harm by using distraction techniques. The recent report from the Mental Health Foundation and the Camelot Foundation (MHF/CF, 2006) suggests that distraction techniques could be an important first step in the client's management of their self-harm.

However, the behaviour is not the most important issue in the care of those who self-harm. What is of most importance is the person behind the behaviour (Zest, 2003, 2006). So how do practitioners get to the person behind the behaviour and what types of therapies are available for those who self-harm? In some cases clients do benefit from the same counselling therapies that are used in attempted suicide but it seems that there is no one size to fit all (MHF/CF, 2006). However, the recent Report of the Inquiry into Self-Harm among Young People (MHF/CF, 2006) cite Fortune, Sinclair and Hawton (2005) as reporting that many young people feel that having someone to listen to them, give them support and advice would help prevent self-harm. It would therefore seem that a minimal therapeutic response would be client-centred therapy as proposed by Rogers (1951, 1961). This would include communicating such qualities as genuineness, non-judgemental attitude, acceptance and respect to the client. This type of caring/therapeutic response to clients who self-harm would convey the practitioner's willingness to engage with them in a genuine and non-judgemental way. In so doing there is a chance that they will respond favourably towards such practitioners. For instance, although it was a small sample, Dunne, Thompson and Leitch (2000) found that adolescent males' experience of counselling was favourable. This finding, in what is known as a difficult group to engage with, bodes well for the future and suggests that using counselling therapies would be beneficial for adolescents experiencing difficulties in their lives. Currently, when it comes to caring for those who self-harm, very little has worked. It seems from research findings that the way care is delivered to those who self-harm is causing clients to feel rejected and abused all over again. It is time that government gave health care authorities the assistance they need to change the way they deliver care to this group who are at very high risk of future suicide.

Summary

This chapter commenced with a look at the medical response to suicide-related behaviour. While medications can be useful, their use in suicide-related behaviour is questionable at other times. There is no pill for every ill. Practitioners need to focus on long-term answers that encourage the client to move back towards a life-orientated position. However, prior to any therapy, whether it is medication or something else, the assessment of the client's need is paramount. The assessment is one of the most important therapeutic interactions with the client. It will involve a set induction and practitioners need to demonstrate skills and qualities that are necessary in a caring practitioner. This is the basis of the therapeutic relationship and if done well it can have a therapeutic effect on the client. In addition, the information gained during the assessment must be made use of; otherwise it will have been a worthless exercise (SCMH, 2006). The assessment can provide insights into a person's risk of future suicide. Also, it can indicate the client's (positive) blind spots and these can help to undermine the client's cognitive distortions.

Alternatives to medications are the counselling therapies. These can help a person work through their crisis and those issues that are causing them despair. In the case of minor to moderate depression, counselling therapies are more useful in the long term than medications. Also, there have been some studies that indicate that psychological therapies such as CBT are somewhat effective in the prevention of suicide-related behaviour (van der Sande et al., 1997). Currently there is a case for making more use of the psychological therapies in the care of those experiencing emotional despair. For instance, the Sainsbury Centre for Mental Health (2006) has reiterated the recommendation by the National Institute for Clinical Excellence (NICE, 2004b) that the psychological therapies must be made available on the NHS. Thus, it seems that pressure is mounting to move away from the current custodial and patriarchal mode of delivering care. Of course this cannot happen overnight and it will require that adequate practitioners are properly trained to deliver the service required. In addition, it will also link independent practitioners, with current statutory services (SCMH, 2006). By actively involving the client in their own treatment, psychological therapies can empower people and encourage them to engage in the process of recovery (SCMH, 2006, p. 13).

In this chapter only one helping model was demonstrated (Egan, 2006) and it briefly introduced the practitioner to how the model works. In addition, cognitive behavioural therapy was also briefly discussed and an outline demonstrated as to how it works. These examples in themselves are informative but they should not replace adequate education and specialist training in counselling. There are other counselling therapies that are useful in helping such as:

1. person-centred therapy
2. gestalt therapy
3. psychoanalytical therapy
4. family systems therapy
5. behaviour therapy
6. reality therapy
7. Adlerian therapy
8. existential therapy.

Obviously, there is inadequate space in this book to cover all of the above therapies. Nonetheless, they are mentioned to show an example of what is available. Therapy is useful but there is no one counselling theory that fits all the requirements and provides all of the answers. However, one theory that can be combined with most is that of Rogers (1951, 1961) client-centred therapy (now called person-centred therapy). This theory may not provide all the answers, but it certainly provides all the caring ingredients that practitioners need to establish a human-to-human connection with a client who is considering suicide-related behaviour. One particular group where practitioners perceive themselves as lacking in competency and where negative attitudes also abound is that of providing care for those who self-harm. The discussion above indicates a way forward for practitioners in caring for these clients. It is suggested that while counselling may eventually be needed, what practitioners have to do in the interim is to demonstrate the core qualities of the helping profession such as empathy, congruence (genuineness), and unconditional positive regard (acceptance). For learners and qualified practitioners alike, these are the essential prerequisites for skilled functioning as practitioners when interacting and helping clients who self-harm or have attempted suicide.

References

Abramson, L., Alloy, L., Hogan, M. *et al.* (1998) Suicidality and cognitive vulnerability to depression among college students: a prospective study. *Journal of Adolescence*, **21**, 473–87.

Adams, J. and Adams, M. (1996) The association among negative life events, perceived problem alternatives, depression, and suicidal ideation in adolescent psychiatric patients. *Journal of Child Psychology and Psychiatry*, **37**, 715–20.

Aguilera, D. (1994) *Crisis Intervention: Theory and Management*, Mosby, St Louis.

Ahrens, B. and Haug, H. (1996) Suicidality in hospitalised patients with a primary diagnosis of personality disorder. *Crisis*, **17** (2), 59–63.

Ajzen, I. (1988) *Attitudes, Personality, and Behavior*, The Dorsey Press, Chicago.

Ajzen, I. (1985) From intentions to actions: a theory of planned behavior, in *Action Control: From Cognition to Behavior* (eds J. Kuhl and J. Beckmann), Springer, Heidelberg.

Ajzen, I. and Timko, C. (1986) Correspondence between health attitudes and behavior. *Basic and Applied Social Psychology*, **7** (4), 259–76.

Altschul, A. (1972) *Patient – Nurse Interaction: A Study of Interactive Patterns in Acute Psychiatric Wards*, Churchill Livingstone, Edinburgh.

Amador, X., Friedman, J., Kasapis, C. *et al.* (1996) Suicidal behaviour in schizophrenia and its relationship to awareness of illness. *American Journal of Psychiatry*, **153** (9), 1185–8.

American Psychiatric Association (2000) *Diagnostic and Statistical Manual of Mental Disorders – Text Revision*, 4th edn (DSM-IV), APA, Washington, DC.

Anderson, M. (1997) Nurses' attitudes towards suicidal behaviour: a comparative study of community mental health nurses and nurses working in an accidents and emergency department. *Journal of Advanced Nursing*, **25** (6), 1283–91.

Anderson, M., Standen, P. and Noon, J. (2003) Nurses' and doctors' perceptions of young people who engage in suicidal behaviour: a contemporary grounded theory analysis. *International Journal of Nursing Studies*, **40** (6), 587–97.

Andrew, B., Hawton, K., Fagg, J. *et al.* (1993) Do psychosocial factors influence outcome in severely depressed female psychiatric in-patients? *British Journal of Psychiatry*, **163**, 747–54.

Andriessen, K. (2006) On 'intention' in the definition of suicide. *Suicide and Life-Threatening Behavior*, **36** (5), 533–8.

Andrus, J., Fleming, D., Heumann, M. *et al.* (1991) Surveillance of attempted suicide in Oregon, 1988. *American Journal of Public Health*, **81** (8), 1067–9.

Anonymous (1990) A nurse in need. *Nursing Times*, **86** (14), 50.

Apter, M.J. (1992) *The Dangerous Edge: The Psychology of Excitement*, Free Press, New York.

Arensman, E. and Kerkhof, A. (1996) Classification of attempted suicide: a review of the empirical studies, 1963–1993. *Suicide and Life-Threatening Behavior*, **26** (1), 46–67.

Arnold, L. (1994) *Understanding Self-Injury*, Bristol Crisis Service for Women, Bristol.

Ashberg, M., Traskman, L. and Thoren, P. (1976) 5 HIAA in the cerebrospinal fluid: a biochemical suicide predictor? *Archives of General Psychiatry*, **33**, 1193–7.

Atha, C., Salkovskis, P. and Storer, D. (1992) Cognitive-behavioural problem solving in the treatment of patients attending a medical emergency department: a controlled trial. *Journal of Psychosomatic Research*, **36** (4), 299–307.

Babiker, G. and Arnold, L. (1997) *The Language of Injury: Comprehending Self-Mutilation*, The British Psychological Press, Leicester.

Badger, T. (1996) Living with depression: family members' experiences and treatment needs. *Journal of Psychosocial and Mental Health Services*, **34** (1), 21–9.

Bailey, S. (1994) Critical care nurses' and doctors' attitudes to parasuicide. *Australian Journal of Advanced Nursing*, **11** (3), 11–17.

Bancroft, J., Skrimshire, A., Casson, J. *et al.* (1977) People who deliberately poison or injure themselves: their problems and their contacts with helping agencies. *Psychological Medicine*, **7**, 289–303.

Bandura, A. (1982) Self-efficacy mechanism in human agency. *American Psychologist*, **37** (2), 122–47.

Bandura, A. (1984) Recycling misconceptions of perceived self-efficacy. *Cognitive Therapy and Research*, **8**, 231–55.

Barbe, R., Bridge, J., Birmaher, B. *et al.* (2004) Suicidality and its relationship to treatment outcome in depressed adolescents. *Suicide and Life-Threatening Behavior*, **34**, 44–55.

Barker, P. (1992) *Severe Depression: A Practitioners Guide*, Chapman & Hall, Glasgow.

Barker, P. (2001) The tidal model: the lived experience in person-centred mental health nursing care. *Nursing Philosophy*, **2** (3), 213–23.

Barker, P. (2003) *Healing the Hurt*. Conference proceedings. City Hotel, Derry, Northern Ireland. October 2003.

Barraclough, B. and Pallis, D. (1975) Depression followed by suicide: a comparison of depressed suicides with living depressives. *Psychological Medicine*, **5**, 55–61.

Barstow, D. (1995) Self-injury and self-mutilation. *Journal of Psychosocial Nursing*, **33**, 19–22.

Beck, A. and Lester, D. (1976) Components of suicide intent in attempted and completed suicide. *Journal of Psychology*, **92**, 35–8.

Beck, A., Kovacs, M. and Weissman, A. (1975) Hopelessness and suicidal behaviour: an overview. *Journal of the American Medical Association*, **234** (11), 1146–9.

Beck, A., Kovacs, M. and Weissman, A. (1979) Assessment of suicidal intent: the scale for suicide ideation. *Journal of Consulting and Clinical Psychology*, **47**, 343–52.

Beck, A., Rush, A., Shaw, B. *et al.* (1979) *Cognitive Therapy of Depression*, Guilford Press, New York.

Beck, A., Schuyler, D. and Herman, I. (1974) Development of suicidal intent scales, in *The Prediction of Suicide* (eds A. Beck, H. Resnik and D. Letteri), Charles Press, Bowie, Maryland, pp. 45–56.

Beck, A., Steer, R., Beck, J. *et al.* (1993) Hopelessness, depression, suicidal ideation and clinical diagnosis of depression. *Suicide and Life-Threatening Behavior*, **29** (2), 139–45.

Beck, A., Steer, R., Kovacs, M. *et al.* (1985) Hopelessness and eventual suicide: a 10-year prospective study of patients hospitalized with suicidal ideation. *American Journal of Psychiatry*, **142** (5), 559–63.

Beck, A., Weissman, A., Lester, D. *et al.* (1974) The Measurement of pessimism: the hopelessness scale. *Journal of Consulting and Clinical Psychology*, **42** (6), 861–5.

Beck, P., Lazarus, J., Scorer, R. *et al.* (1994) Increasing rate of deliberate self-poisoning. *British Medical Journal*, **308**, 789.

Bentley, J. (1988) Body language: non-verbal communication and the nurse. *Nursing Standard*, **2** (36), 30–2.

Blair, D. (1996) Integration and synthesis: cognitive behavioral therapies within the biological paradigm. *Journal of Psychosocial Nursing and Mental Health Services*, **34** (12), 26–31.

Blaney, R. and MacKenzie, G. (1978) *A Northern Ireland Community Health Study*, Department of Community Medicine, Queen's University of Belfast, Belfast.

Boldero, J. and Fallon, B. (1995) Adolescent help-seeking: what do they get and from whom? *Journal of Adolescence*, **18** (2), 193–209.

Bolland, J. (2003) Hopelessness and risk behaviour among adolescents living in high-poverty inner-city neighbourhoods. *Journal of Adolescence*, **26**, 145–58.

Bone, V. (2005) Dad kills himself after his son and daughter commit suicide. *Daily Mirror*, 21 December, p. 29.

Bowers, L., Gournay, K. and Duffy, D. (2000) Suicide and self-harm in inpatient psychiatric units: a national survey of observation policies. *Journal of Advanced Nursing*, **32** (2), 437–44.

Bowler, N. (2001) Suicide and social exclusion in Wales. *Mental Health Nursing*, **21** (3), 6–9.

Bowles, N., Dodds, P., Hackney, D. *et al.* (2002) Formal observations and engagements: a discussion paper. *Journal of Psychiatric and Mental Health Nursing*, **9**, 255–60.

Boyd, J. and Weissman, M. (1982) Epidemiology, in *Handbook of Affective Disorders* (ed. E.S. Paykel), Churchill Livingstone, Edinburgh, pp. 109–25.

Bradshaw, J. (1988) *Bradshaw: On the Family. A Revolutionary Way of Self-Discovery*, Health Communications Inc., Deerfield Beach, Florida.

Bradshaw, J. (1996) *Bradshaw: On the Family. A New Way of Creating Solid Self-Esteem*, Health Communications Inc., Deerfield Beach, Florida.

Brent, D., Perper, J., Goldstein, C. *et al.* (1988) Risk factors for adolescents: a comparison of adolescent suicide victims with suicidal inpatients. *Archives of General Psychiatry*, **45**, 581–8.

Brodsky, B., Oquendo, M., Ellis, S. *et al.* (2001) The relationship of childhood abuse to impulsivity and suicidal behavior in adults with major depression. *American Journal of Psychiatry*, **158**, 1871–7.

Brookshank, D. (1985) Suicide and parasuicide in childhood and early adolescence. *British Journal of Psychiatry*, **146**, 459–63.

Brown, G.L., Goodwin, F.K., Ballenger, J.C. *et al.* (1979) Aggression in humans correlates with cerebrospinal amine metabolites. *Psychiatry Research*, **1**, 131–9.

Brown, G.W. and Harris, T. (1978) *The Social Origins of Depression*, Tavistock Publications, London.

Brádvik, L. (2003) Suicide after suicide attempt in severe depression; A long-term follow-up. *Suicide and Life-Threatening Behavior*, **33** (4), 381–8.

Burgess, S., Hawton, K. and Loveday, G. (1998) Adolescents who take overdoses: outcomes in terms of changes in psychopathology and the adolescents' attitude to care and to their overdose. *Journal of Adolescence*, **21**, 209–18.

Burvill, P., McCall, M., Woodings, T. and Stenhouse, N. (1983) Comparison of suicide rates and methods in English, Scots, and Irish migrants in Australia. *Social Science Medicine*, **17**, 705–8.

Buston, K. (2002) Adolescents with mental health problems: what do they say about health services? *Journal of Adolescence*, **25**, 231–42.

Cannon, W. (1929) *Bodily Changes in Pain, Hunger, Fear and Rage*, 2nd edn, Appleton, New York.

Caplan, G. (1964) *An Approach to Community Mental Health*, Tavistock, London.

Carlton, P. and Deane, F. (2000) Impact of attitudes and suicidal ideation on adolescents' intentions to seek professional psychological help. *Journal of Adolescence*, **23**, 35–45.

Carrigan, J. (1994) The psychosocial needs of patients who have attempted suicide by overdose. *Journal of Advanced Nursing*, **20** (4), 635–42.

Carveth, J. (1995) Perceived patient deviance and avoidance by nurses. *Nursing Research*, **44** (3), 173–8.

van Casteren, V., VanderVeken, J., Tafforeau, J. *et al.* (1993) Suicide and attempted suicide reported by general practitioners in Belgium. *Acta Psychiatrica Scandinavica*, **87** (6), 451–5.

Castillo, H., Allen, L. and Coxhead, N. (2001) The hurtfulness of a diagnosis; User research about personality disorder. *Mental Health Practice*, **4** (9), 16–19.

Catalan, J. (1983) Attempted suicide and homosexuality. *British Journal of Sexual Medicine*, **20**, 11–14.

Catalan, J. and Gath, D. (1985) Benzodiazapines in general practice: time for a decision. *British Medical Journal*, **290**, 1374–6.

Catalan, J., Gath, D., Edmonds, G. and Ennis, J. (1984a) The effects of non-prescribing of anxiolytics in a general practice – 1: controlled evaluation of psychiatric and social outcome. *British Journal of Psychiatry*, **144**, 593–602.

Catalan, J., Gath, D., Bond, A. and Martin, P. (1984b) The effects of non-prescribing of anxiolytics in a general practice – II: factors associated with outcome. *British Journal of Psychiatry*, **144**, 603–10.

Catalan, J., Marsack, P., Hawton, K. *et al.* (1980a) Comparison of doctors and nurses in the assessment of deliberate self-poisoning patients. *Psychological Medicine*, **10**, 483–91.

Catalan, J., Hewett, J., Kennard, C. and McPherson, J. (1980b) The role of the nurse in the management of deliberate self-poisoning in the general hospital. *International Journal of Nursing Studies*, **17** (4), 275–82.

Champion, L., Goodall, G. and Rutter, M. (1995) Behaviour problems in childhood and stressors in early adult life: 1. A 20-year follow-up of London school children. *Psychological Medicine*, **25** (2), 231–46.

Chapman, J. (2005) *Daily Express* (UK), 12 February 2005, p. 37.

Chatterton, R. (1995) Parasuicide in people with schizophrenia. *Australian and New Zealand Journal of Mental Health Nursing*, **4** (2), 83–6.

Cheng, A. (1995) Mental illness and suicide. *Archives of General Psychiatry*, **52**, 594–603.

Chin, M.A., Touquet, R. and Burns, T. (1986) Contact of parasuicide patients with the accident and emergency department. *Archives of Emergency Medicine*, **3** (3), 177–82.

Clark, D. and Fawcett, J. (1992) Review of empirical risk factors for evaluation of the suicidal patient, in *Suicide: Guidelines for Assessment, Management, and Treatment* (ed. B. Bongar), Oxford University Press, Oxford, pp. 16–48.

Coccaro, E.F. (1992) Impulsive aggression and central serotonergic system functions in humans: an example of a dimensional brain-behaviour relationship. *International Clinical Psychopharmacology*, **7**, 3–12.

Cohen, S. and Herbert, T. (1996) Health psychology: psychological factors and physical disease from the perspective of human psychoneuroimmunology. *Annual Review of Psychology*, **47**, 113–23.

Cohen, S. and Wills, T. (1985) Stress, social support and the buffering hypothesis. *Psychological Bulletin*, **98**, 310–57.

Connors, R. (1996) Self-Injury in trauma survivors: 1. Functions and meanings. *American Journal of Orthopsychiatry*, **66**, 197–206.

Conrad, N. (1991) Where do they turn to? Social support systems of suicidal high school adolescents. *Journal of Psychosocial Nursing and Mental Health Services*, **29** (3), 14–20.

Conrad, N. (1992) Stress and knowledge of suicidal others as factors in suicidal behaviour of high school adolescents. *Issues in Mental Health Nursing*, **13** (2), 95–104.

Cooper, J., Kapur, N., Webb, R. *et al.* (2005) Suicide after deliberate self-harm: a 4 year cohort study. *American journal of psychiatry*, **162**, 297–303.

Corey, G. (2005) *Theory and Practice of Counseling & Psychotherapy*, 7th edn, Brooks/Cole, Belmont, CA.

Crawford, T., Geraghty, W., Street, K. and Simonoff, E. (2003) Staff knowledge and attitudes towards deliberate self-harm in adolescents. *Journal of Adolescence*, **26** (5), 623–33.

Cremniter, D., Jamain, S., Kollenbach, K. *et al.* (1999) CSF 5-HIAA levels are lower in impulsive as compared to non-impulsive violent suicide attempters and control subjects. *Biological Psychiatry*, **45**, 1572–9.

Crockett, A. (1987) Patterns of consultation and parasuicide. *British Medical Journal of Clinical Research*, **295**, 476–8.

Cummings, A., Slemon, A. and Hallberg, E. (1993) Session evaluation and recall of important events as a function of counselor experience. *Journal of Counseling Psychology*, **40**, 156–65.

D'Augelli, A. and Hershberger, S. (1993) Gay and bisexual youth in community settings: personal challenges and mental health problems. *American Journal of Community Psychology*, **21**, 421–48.

Davidson, J., Hughes, D., George, L. *et al.* (1996) The association of sexual assault and attempted suicide within the community. *Archives of General Psychiatry*, **53** (6), 550–5.

Dawson, P. (1997) A Reply to Kevin Gournay's schizophrenia: a review of the contemporary literature and implications for mental health nursing theory, practice and education. *Journal of Psychiatric and Mental Health Nursing*, **4** (1), 1–7.

De La Fuente, R. (1990) The mental health consequences of the 1985 earthquakes in Mexico. *International Journal of Mental Health*, **19**, 21–9.

De Moore, G.M. and Robertson, A.R. (1996) Risk factors for suicide in deliberate self-harm. *British Journal of Psychiatry*, **169**, 489–94.

De Wilde, E., Kienhorst, C., Diekstra, R. *et al.* (1994) Social support, life events and behavioral characteristics of psychologically distressed adolescents at high risk for attempting suicide. *Adolescence*, **29** (113), 49–60.

Dear, G. (1997) Letter to the editor. Writing this was instrumental, whatever my intent: a comment. *Suicide and Life-Threatening Behavior*, **27** (4), 408–10.

Deffenbacher, J. (1996) Cognitive-behavioral approaches to anger reduction, in *Advances in Cognitive-Behavioral Therapy* (eds K. Dobson and K. Craig), Sage Publications, New Delhi.

Dennis, M., Owens, D. and Jones, S. (1990) Epidemiology of deliberate self-poisoning trends in hospital attendances. *Health Trends*, **22**, 125–6.

Department of Health (1993) *The Health of the Nation: A Contact for Health*, HMSO, London.

Department of Health (2001) *Safety First: Five-Year Report of the National Confidential Inquiry into Suicide and Homicide by People with Mental Illness*, HMSO, London.

Department of Health and Social Security (1984) *The Management of Deliberate Self-Harm. HN(84)25*, HMSO, London.

Department of Health and the Home Office (1994) *Report of the Department of Health and Home Office Working Group on Psychopathetic Disorder*, HMSO, London.

Department of Health, Social Services and Public Safety Northern Ireland (2006) *Protect Life: A Shared Vision. The Northern Ireland Suicide Prevention Strategy and Action Plan 2006-2011 – A Consultation Document*, DHSSPSNI, Belfast.

Dickinson, G., Lancaster, C., Clark, D. *et al.* (2002) U.K. physicians' attitudes toward active voluntary euthanasia and physician-assisted suicide. *Death studies*, **26** (6), 479–90.

Diekstra, R. (1986) The significance of Nico Speijer's suicide. How and when should suicide be prevented? *Suicide and Life-Threatening Behaviour*, **16**, 13–15.

Diekstra, R. and Van Egmond, M. (1989) Suicide and attempted suicide in general practice: 1979–1986. *Acta Psychiatrica Scandinavica*, **79**, 268–75.

Dobson, K. and Jackman-Cram, S. (1996) Common change processes in cognitive-behavioral therapies for depression, in *Advances in Cognitive-Behavioral Therapy* (eds K. Dobson and K. Craig), Sage Publications, New Delhi.

Dorer, C., Feehan, C., Vostanis, P. *et al.* (1999) The overdose process – adolescents' experience of taking an overdose and their contact with services. *Journal of Adolescence*, **22**, 413–17.

Drake, R. and Cotton, P. (1986) Depression, hopelessness, and suicide in chronic schizophrenia. *British Journal of Psychiatry*, **148**, 554–9.

Duffield, B. (1992) The perpetual shadow. *Nursing Times*, **88** (23), 28–9.

Duffy, D. (1995) Out of the Shadows: a study of the special observation of suicidal psychiatric in-patients. *Journal of Advanced Nursing*, **21** (5), 944–50.

Dunham, K. (2004) Young adults' support strategies when peers disclose suicidal intent. *Suicide and Life-Threatening Behaviour*, **34** (1), 56–65.

Dunleavey, R. (1992) An adequate response to a cry for help? Parasuicide patients' perceptions of their nursing care. *Professional Nurse*, **7** (4), 213–15.

Dunne, A., Thompson, W. and Leitch, R. (2000) Adolescent males' experience of the counselling process. *Journal of Adolescence*, **23**, 79–93.

Durkheim, E. (1897/1951) *Suicide: A Study in Sociology*, Translation by J.A. Spaulding (1951), Routledge & Kegan Paul, London.

Eastwick, Z. and Grant, A. (2004) Emotional rescue: deliberate self harmers and A&E departments. *Mental Health Nursing Practice*, **7** (9), 12–15.

Egan, G. (2006) *The Skilled Helper: A Problem-Management and Opportunity-Development Approach to Helping*, 8th edn, Brooks/Cole, Pacific Grove, California.

van Egmond, M. and Diekstra, R. (1990) The predictability of suicidal behavior: the results of a meta-analysis of published studies. *Crisis*, **11** (2), 57–84.

van Egmond, M., Garnefski, N., Jonker, D. *et al.* (1993) The relationship between sexual abuse and female suicidal behaviour. *Crisis*, **14** (3), 129–39.

Elliott, R. and Wexler, M. (1994) Measuring the impact of sessions in process experimental-therapy of depression: the sessions impact scale. *Journal of Counseling Psychology*, **41**, 166–74.

Ellis, T. (1988) Classification of suicidal behaviour: a review and step towards integration. *Suicide and Life-Threatening Behaviour*, **18** (4), 358–71.

Erikson, E. (1977) *Childhood and Society*, Paladin, London.

Erikson, E. (1985) *The Life Cycle Completed: A Review*, Norton, New York.

Essinger, D. (2003) Attitudes of Tennessee physicians toward euthanasia and assisted death. *Southern Medical Journal*, **96** (5), 427–35.

Evans, M. (1994) Using a psychoanalytic model to approach acts of self-harm. *Nursing Times*, **90** (42), 38–40.

Evans, M., Cox, C. and Turnball, G. (1992) Parasuicide response. *Nursing Times*, **88** (19), 34–6.

Farmer, R. and Creed, F. (1989) Life events and hostility in self-poisoning. *British Journal of Psychiatry*, **154**, 390–5.

Fennell, M. (1989) Depression, in *Cognitive Behaviour Therapy for Psychiatric Problems* (eds K. Hawton, P. Salkovskis, J. Kirk and D. Clark), Oxford University Press, Oxford.

Fitzpatrick, J., Whall, A., Johnston, R. *et al.* (1982) *Nursing Models and Their Psychiatric Mental Health Applications*, Prentice Hall, London.

Food and Drug Administration (US) (2004) FDA Public Health Advisory: worsening depression and suicidality in patients being treated with antidepressant. 22 March 2004. http://www.fda.gov.cder/drug/antidepressants/AntidepressanstPHA.htm (20 December 2006).

Food and Drug Administration (US) (2005) FDA Public Health Advisory: Suicidality in Adults being treated with antidepressant medications. 30 June 2005. http://www.fda.gov.cder/drug/advisory/SSRI200507.htm (20 December 2006).

Fortune, S., Sinclair, J. and Hawton, K. (2005) *Adolescents Views on the Prevention of Self-Harm, Barriers to Help-Seeking for Self-Harm and how Quality of Life Can Be Improved: A Qualitative and Quantitative Study*, Centre for suicide research, University of Oxford, Oxford.

Foster, T., Gillespie, K. and McClelland, R. (1997) Mental disorders and suicide in Northern Ireland. *British Journal of Psychiatry*, **170**, 447–52.

Free, M., Oei, T. and Sanders, M. (1991) Treatment outcome of a group cognitive therapy programme for depression. *International Journal of Group Psychotherapy*, **41**, 533–47.

Fremouw, W., Callahan, T. and Kashden, J. (1993) Adolescent suicidal risk: psychological, problem solving, and environmental factors. *Suicide and Life-Threatening Behaviour*, **23** (1), 46–54.

Freud, S. (1900/1953) *The Interpretation of Dreams* (Reprint Edition, Vol. 4, 5), Hogarth Press, London (Original work published in 1900).

Freud, S. (1905/1977) *Three Essays on the Theory of Sexuality*, Penguin, Hammondsworth, Middlesex (Original work published in 1905).

Freud, S. (1917/1957) Mourning and melancholia, in *The Standard Edition of the Complete Psychological Works of Sigmund Freud* (ed. J. Strahy), Hogarth Press, London, pp. 209–18.

Freud, S. (1922/1984) *Beyond the Pleasure Principle. Pelican Freud Library (11)*. Penguin, Hammondsworth, Middlesex (Original work published in 1922).

Freud, S. (1940) An outline of psychoanalysis. *International Journal of Psychoanalysis*, **21**, 27–84.

Friedman, R.C. and Corn, R. (1985) Follow-Up five years after attempted suicide at age 7. *American Journal of Psychotherapy*, **39** (1), 108–13.

Friedman, T., Newton, C., Coggan, C. *et al.* (2006) Predictors of A&E staff attitudes to self-harm patients who use self-laceration: influence of previous training and experience. *Journal of Psychosomatic Research*, **60** (3), 273–7.

Galloway, D. (ed.) (1967) *A Descent into the Maelström*, Selected Writings of Edgar Allan Poe, Penguin Books, Baltimore, Maryland.

Gibbs, A. (1990) Aspects of communication with people who have attempted suicide. *Journal of Advanced Nursing*, **15** (11), 1245–9.

Gillman, V. and Wilson, J. (1996) Rights and responsibilities: suicide and the decision to die. *Mental Health Nursing*, **16** (3), 7.

Ginn, P.D., Range, L.M. and Hailey, B.J. (1988) Community attitudes towards childhood suicide and attempted suicide. *Journal of Community Psychology*, **16** (2), 144–51.

Gladstone, G., Parker, G., Mitchell, P. *et al.* (2004) Implications of childhood trauma for depressed women: an analysis of pathways from childhood sexual abuse to deliberate self-harm and revictimization. *American Journal of Psychiatry*, **161**, 1417–25.

Goldney, R. and Bottrill, A. (1980) Attitudes towards patients who attempt suicide. *Medical Journal of Australia*, **2** (13), 717–20.

Goldney, R., Winefield, A., Tiggerman, M. *et al.* (1989) Suicidal ideation in a young adult population. *Acta Psychiatricia Scandinavica*, **79**, 481–9.

Goleman, D. (2006) *Emotional Intelligence: Why It Can Matter More than IQ*, Bantam Book, New York.

Gould, M., Fisher, P., Parides, M. *et al.* (1996) Psychosocial risk factors and adolescent completed suicide. *Archives of General Psychiatry*, **53** (12), 1155–62.

Greenblath, M., Becarra, R. and Serafetinides, M. (1982) Social networks and mental health: an overview. *American Journal of Psychiatry*, **139** (8), 977–84.

Gunnell, D., Peters, T., Kammerling, R. *et al.* (1995) Relation between parasuicide, suicide, psychiatric admissions and socioeconomic deprivation. *British Medical Journal*, **311** (6999), 226–30.

Homefirst Community Trust (1997) *Young Peoples' Health and Social Needs in the Northern Health and Social Services Board Area*, Northern Health and Social Services Board, Ballymena, Northern Ireland.

Haaga, D., Dyck, M. and Ernst, D. (1991) Empirical status of cognitive theory of depression. *Psychological Bulletin*, **110**, 215–36.

Handwerk, M., Larzelere, R., Friman, P. *et al.* (1998) The relationship between lethality of attempted suicide and prior communications in a sample of residential youth. *Journal of Adolescence*, **21**, 407–14.

Hargie, O. and Dickson, D. (2004) *Skilled Interpersonal Communication: Research, Theory and Practice*, 4th edn, Routeledge, New York.

Harkavy-Friedman, J., Nelson, E., Venarde, D. and Mann, J. (2004) Suicidal behavior in schizophrenia and schizoaffective disorder: examining the role of depression. *Suicide and Life-Threatening Behaviour*, **34** (1), 66–76.

Harris, J. (2000) Self harm: cutting the bad out of me. *Qualitative Health Research*, **10** (2), 164–73.

Haw, C., Hawton, K., Houston, K. and Townsend, E. (2003) Correlates of relative lethality and suicidal intent among deliberate self-harm patients. *Suicide and Life-Threatening Behaviour*, **33** (4), 353–64.

Haw, C., Hawton, K., Sutton, L. *et al.* (2005) Schizophrenia and deliberate self-harm: a systematic review of risk factors. *Suicide and Life-Threatening Behaviour*, **35** (1), 50–62.

Hawton, K. (1982) Attempted suicide in children and adolescents. *Journal of Child Psychology and Psychiatry*, **23** (4), 497–503.

Hawton, K. (1991) Repetition and suicide following attempted suicide, in *Current Approaches: Suicide and Attempted Suicide Risk Factors, Management and Prevention* (eds S. Montgomery and N. Goeting), Duphar Laboratories Southampton, pp. 34–40.

Hawton, K. (1993) By their own hand: suicide is increasing in young men. *British Medical Journal*, **304**, 1000.

Hawton, K. (1994a) Adolescent suicide and attempted suicide: the importance of substance abuse. *Crisis*, **15** (1), 8, 13–14.

Hawton, K. (1994b) Youth suicide: trends indicate increasing hopelessness in young males. *Crisis*, **15** (4), 159–60, 163.

Hawton, K. (2002) United Kingdom legislation on pack sizes of analgesics: background, rationale, and effects of suicide and deliberate self-harm. *Suicide and Life-Threatening Behavior*, **32** (3), 223–9.

Hawton, K. and Blackstock, E. (1976) General practice aspects of self-poisoning and self-injury. *Psychological Medicine*, **6**, 571–5.

Hawton, K. and Catalan, J. (1987) *Attempted Suicide: A Practical Guide to Its Nature and Management*, 2nd edn, Oxford University Press, New York.

Hawton, K. and Fagg, J. (1992) Deliberate self-poisoning and self-injury in adolescents: a study of characteristics and trends in Oxford, 1976 – 1989. *British Journal of Psychiatry*, **161**, 816–23.

Hawton, K., Bancroft, J. and Simkin, S. (1978) Attitudes of psychiatric patients to deliberate self-poisoning. *British Journal of Psychiatry*, **132**, 31–5.

Hawton, K., Fagg, J. and McKeown, S. (1989) Alcoholism, alcohol, and attempted suicide. *Alcohol and Alcoholism*, **24** (1), 3–9.

Hawton, K., Fagg, J., Simkim, S. *et al.* (2000) Deliberate self-harm in adolescents in Oxford, 1985–1995. *Journal of Adolescence*, **23**, 47–55.

Hawton, K., Fagg, J. and Simkin, S. (1988) Female unemployment and attempted suicide. *British Journal of Psychiatry*, **152**, 632–7.

Hawton, K., Fagg, J. and Simkin, S. (1996) Deliberate self-poisoning and self-injury in children and adolescents under 16 years of age in Oxford, 1976–1993. *British Journal of Psychiatry*, **169**, 202–8.

Hawton, K., Haigh, R., Simkin, S. *et al.* (1995) Attempted suicide in Oxford University students, 1976–1990. *Psychological Medicine*, **25**, 179–88.

Hawton, K., Harriss, L., Bale, E. and Bond, A. (2004) Self-cutting: patient characteristics compared with self-poisoners. *Suicide and Life-Threatening Behavior*, **34** (3), 199–208.

Hawton, K., Marsack, P. and Fagg, J. (1981) The attitudes of psychiatrists to deliberate self-poisoning: comparison with physicians and nurses. *British Journal of Medical Psychology*, **54**, 341–8.

Hawton, K., O'Grady, J., Osborn, M. *et al.* (1982) Adolescents who take overdoses: their characteristics, problems and contact with helping agencies. *British Journal of Psychiatry*, **140**, 118–23.

Hawton, K., Rodham, K., Evans, E. and Weatherall, R. (2002) Deliberate self-harm in adolescents: self report survey in schools in England. *British Medical Journal*, **325**, 1207–11.

Health Promotion Agency for Northern Ireland (2002) *Adult Drinking Patterns in Northern Ireland*, Health Promotion Agency, Belfast.

Health Promotion Agency for Northern Ireland (2003) *Attitudes and Behaviour of Young Adult Drinkers in Northern Ireland*, Health Promotion Agency, Belfast.

Health Service Executive (2005) *Reach Out: National Strategy for Action on Suicide Prevention*, HSE, Dublin.

Heikkinen, M., Aro, H. and Lonnqvist, J. (1993) Life events and social support in suicide. *Suicide and Life-Threatening Behavior*, **23**, 343–58.

Hemmings, A. (1999) Attitudes to deliberate self-harm among staff in an accident and emergency team. *Mental Health Care*, **2**, 300–2.

Higley, J., Mehlman, P., Taub, D. *et al.* (1993) Paternal and maternal genetic and environmental contributions to CSF monoamine metabolite concentration in rhesus monkeys. *Archives of General Psychiatry*, **50**, 615–23.

Hjelmeland, H., Nordvik, H., Brahe-Bille, U. *et al.* (2000) A cross-cultural study of suicide intent in parasuicide patients. *Suicide and Life-Threatening Behavior*, **30** (4), 295–303.

Holmes, T. and Rahe, R. (1967) The social readjustment rating scale. *Journal of Psychosomatic Research*, **11**, 213–18.

Information Analysis Directorate (2006) *Section 75 Analysis of Suicide and Self-harm in Northern Ireland (2000–2005)*, DHSSPSNI, Belfast.

Institute for Public Policy Research (2006) Freedom's orphans: raising youth in a changing world. http://www.ippr.org/publicationsandreports/ (6 November 2006).

Isometsa, E. and Lonnqvist, J. (1998) Suicide attempts preceding completed suicide. *British Journal of Psychiatry*, **173**, 531–5.

Jahoda, M. (1958) *Current Concepts of Positive Mental Health*, Basic Books Publishers, New York.

James, D. and Hawton, K. (1985) Overdoses: explanations and attitudes in self-poisoners and significant others. *British Journal of Psychiatry*, **146**, 481–5.

Jeffrey, D. and Warm, A. (2002) A study of service providers' understanding of self harm. *Journal of Mental Health*, **11** (3), 295–303.

Jianlin, J. (1993) Crisis intervention for attempted suicide in Shanghai, China. *Stress Medicine*, **9** (2), 87–9.

Johnsson Fridell, E., Ojehagen, A. and Traskman-Bendz, L. (1996) A 5-Year follow-up study of suicide attempts. *Acta Scandinavica Psychiatrica*, **93** (3), 151–7.

Johnstone, L. (1997) Self-injury and the psychiatric response. *Feminism and Psychology*, **7**, 421–6.

Jones, A. (1996) An equal struggle (psychodynamic assessment following repeated episodes of deliberate self-harm). *Journal of Psychiatric and Mental Health Nursing*, **3** (3), 173–80.

Kalisch, B. (1973) What is empathy? *American Journal of Nursing*, **73** (9), 1548–52.

Kanner, A. and Feldman, S. (1991) Control over uplifts and hassles and its relationship to adaptational outcomes. *Journal of Behavioural Medicine*, **4**, 1–39.

Keir, N. (1986) *I Can't Face Tomorrow*, Thornsons, Rochester.

Kelleher, M., Keohane, B., Corcoran, P. *et al.* (2000) An investigation of one hundred suicides. *Iris Journal of Psychological Medicine*, **17** (3), 86–90.

Kerfoot, M., Dyer, E., Harrington, V. *et al.* (1996) Correlates and short-term course of self-poisoning in adolescents. *British Journal of Psychiatry*, **168**, 38–42.

Kessler, R., Borges, G. and Walters, E. (1999) Prevalence of and risk factors for lifetime suicide attempts in the National Comorbidity Survey. *Archives of General Psychiatry*, **56**, 617–26.

Kevorkian, J. (1991) *Prescription Medicine: The Goodness of Planned Death*, Prometheus Books, Buffalo, NY.

King, E. (1994) Suicide in the mentally ill: an epidemiological sample and implications for clinicians. *British Journal of Psychiatry*, **165** (5), 658–63.

Kipling, R. (1902) The elephant child, in *Just So Stories* (ed. R. Kipling), Macmillan, London.

Kitchener, B. and Jorm, A. (2002) *Mental Health First Aid Program*, ORYGEN Research Centre, University of Melbourne.

Klerman, G. (1987) Clinical epidemiology of suicide. *Journal of Clinical Psychiatry*, **48** (12), 33–8.

Kobasa, S., Hilker, R. and Maddi, S. (1979) Psychological hardiness. *Journal of Occupational Medicine*, **21**, 595–8.

Kreitman, N. (ed.) (1977) *Parasuicide*, John Wiley & Sons, Inc., London.

Kreitman, N. (1989) Can suicide and parasuicide be prevented? *Journal of the Royal Society of Medicine*, **82** (11), 648–52.

Kreitman, N. and Casey, P. (1988) Repetition of parasuicide: an epidemiological and clinical study. *British Journal of Psychiatry*, **153**, 792–800.

Kreitman, N. and Chowdhury, N. (1973) Distress behaviour: a study of selected samaritan clients and parasuicides (attempted suicide patients). *British Journal of Psychiatry*, **123**, 1–14.

Kreitman, N., Philip, A., Greer, S. *et al.* (1969) Parasuicide. *British Journal of Psychiatry*, **115**, 746–7.

Kulik, J. and Mahler, H. (1993) Emotional support as a moderator of adjustment and compliance after coronary artery bypass surgery: a longitudinal study. *Journal of Behavioural Medicine*, **16**, 45–54.

La Piere, R. (1934) Attitudes versus actions. *Social Forces*, **13**, 230–7.

Lam, D. (1997) Cognitive behaviour therapy territory model: effective disputing approach. *Journal of Advanced Nursing*, **25** (6), 1205–9.

Lawlor, M. and James, D. (2000) Prevalence of psychological problems in Irish school going adolescents. *Irish Journal of Psychological Medicine*, **17** (4), 117–22.

Lazarus, R. (1981) Little hassles can be hazardous to health. *Psychology Today*, **15**, 58–62.

Lazarus, R. (1993) Coping theory and research: past, present, and future. *Psychosomatic Medicine*, **55**, 234–47.

Lazarus, R. and Folkman, S. (1984) *Stress, Appraisal, and Coping*, Springer, New York.

Leenaars, A. and Connolly, J. (2001) Suicide, assisted suicide and euthanasia: international perspectives. *Irish Journal of Psychological Medicine*, **18** (1), 33–7.

Leonard, C. (1967) *Understanding and Preventing Suicide*, Charles C. Thomas, Illinois.

Levine, J. (2005) *Sunday World* (UK), 13 February 2005, p. 43.

Leyens, J. and Codol, J. (1988) Social cognition, in *Introduction to Social Psychology* (eds M. Hewstone, W. Strobbe, J. Codol and M. Stephenson), Basil Blackwell Ltd., Oxford, pp. 89–110.

Libberton, P. (1996) Depressed and suicidal clients: how nurses can help. *Nursing Times*, **92** (43), 38–40.

Lindgren, B., Wilstand, C., Gilje, F. and Olofsson, B. (2004) Struggling for hopefulness: a qualitative study of Swedish women who self-harm. *Journal of Psychiatric and Mental Health Nursing*, **11**, 284–91.

Linehan, M., Camper, P., Chiles, J. *et al.* (1987) Interpersonal problem solving and parasuicide. *Cognitive Therapy and Research*, **11** (1), 1–12.

LivingWorks (2004) *Suicide Intervention Handbook*, LivingWorks Education Inc., Calgary, Alberta.

Long, A. and Reid, W. (1996) An exploration of nurses' attitudes to the nursing care of the suicidal patient in an acute psychiatric ward. *Journal of Psychiatric and Mental Health Nursing*, **3** (1), 29–37.

Lovett, C. and Maltsberger, J. (1992) Psychodynamic approaches to the assessment and management of suicide, in *Suicide: Guidelines for Assessment, Management, and Treatment* (ed. B. Bongar), Oxford University Press, Oxford, pp. 160–75.

Luft, J. and Ingham, H. (1963) The Johari Window: a graphic model of awareness in interpersonal relations, in *Group Processes: An Introduction to Group Dynamics* (ed. J. Luft), National Press, Palo Alto, California, pp. 10–12.

Lynch, T. (2005) *Beyond Prozac: helping mental distress*, Mercier Press Ltd, Cork.

Lynn, F. (1998) The pain of rejection. *Nursing Times*, **94** (27), 36.

McAllister, M. and Estefan, A. (2002) Principles and strategies for teaching therapeutic responses to self-harm. *Journal of Psychiatric and Mental Health Nursing*, **9**, 573–83.

McAllister, M., Creedy, D., Moyle, W. and Farrugia, C. (2002) Nurses' attitudes towards clients who self-harm. *Journal of Advanced Nursing*, **40** (5), 578–86.

McCann, T., Clark, E., McConnachie, S. and Harvey, I. (2006) Accident and emergency nurses's attitudes towards patients who self-harm. *Accident Emergency Nursing*, **14** (1), 4–10.

McGlashan, T. (1984) The chestnut lodge follow-up study, part ii: long-term outcome of schizophrenia and the affective disorders. *Archives of General Psychiatry*, **41**, 586–601.

McGonagle, I. and Gentle, J. (1996) Reasons for non-attendance at a day hospital for people with enduring mental illness: the clients' perspective. *Journal of Psychiatric and Mental Health Nursing*, **3** (1), 61–6.

Mackay, N. and Barrowclough, C. (2005) Accident and emergency staffs' perceptions of deliberate self-harm: attributions, emotions and willingness to help. *British Journal of Clinical Psychology*, **44**, 255–67.

Mackinnon, L. (2005) *Daily Record* (UK), 19 September, pp. 1, 4–5.

McLaughlin, C. (1994) Casualty nurses' attitudes to attempted suicide. *Journal of Advanced Nursing*, **20**, 1111–18.

McLaughlin, C. (1995) Counselling the overdose patient in casualty. *British Journal of Nursing*, **4** (12), 688–90, 707–8.

McLaughlin, J.F.C. (1997a) Psychiatric nurses psychotherapeutic communications with suicidal patients. Unpublished PhD Thesis. Coleraine Campus: University of Ulster.

McLaughlin, C. (1997b) Student nurses' attitudes to the mentally ill: the effect of classroom theory and contact with patients. *Journal of Advanced Nursing*, **26** (6), 1221–8.

McLaughlin, C. (1999) An exploration of psychiatric nurses' and patients' opinions regarding in-patient care for suicidal patients. *Journal of Advanced Nursing*, **29** (5), 1042–51.

McLaughlin, C. and Whittington, D. (1996) Suicide in Northern Ireland: a comparison of two quinquennia (1982–1986 and 1987–1991). *Journal of Psychiatric and Mental Health Nursing*, **3** (1), 13–20.

McLaughlin, J.A., Miller, P. and Warwick, H. (1996) Deliberate self-harm in adolescents: hopelessness, depression, problems and problem-solving. *Journal of Adolescence*, **19**, 523–32.

MacLeod, A., Rose, G. and Williams, J. (1993) Components of hopelessness about the future in parasuicide. *Cognitive Therapy and Research*, **17** (5), 441–55.

McLeod, J. (1991) Childhood parental loss and adult depression. *Journal of Health and Social Behaviour*, **32**, 205–20.

Mahoney, M. (1974) *Cognition and Behavior Modification*, Ballinger, Cambridge, MA.

Malone, K., Haas, G., Sweeney, J. *et al.* (1995) Major depression and the risk of attempted suicide. *Journal of Affective Disorders*, **34** (3), 173–85.

Mann, J., Waternaux, C., Hass, G. and Malone, K. (1999) Toward a clinical model of suicidal behaviour in psychiatric patients. *American Journal of Psychiatry*, **156**, 181–9.

Marchetto, M. (2006) Repetitive skin-cutting: parental bonding, personality and gender. Psychology and psychotherapy: theory. *Research and Practice*, **79** (3), 445–59.

Maris, R., Berman, A. and Silverman, M. (2000) *Comprehensive Textbook of Suicidology*, The Guilford Press, New York.

Meek, C. (2004) Antidepressants. Health which? Consumers Association. February 2004, 22–5.

Mehlmann, P., Higley, J., Faucher, I. *et al.* (1994) Low CSF 5-HIAA concentrations and severe aggression and impaired impulse control in nonhuman primates. *American Journal of Psychiatry*, **151**, 1485–91.

Meichenbaum, D. (1977) *Cognitive-Behavior Modification: An Integrative Approach*, Plenum Press, New York.

Meissner, W. (1977) Psychoanalytic notes on suicide. *International Journal of Psychoanalytic Psychotherapy*, **6**, 415–47.

Mendonca, J. and Holden, R. (1996) Are all suicidal ideas closely linked to hopelessness? *Acta Psychiatrica Scandinavica*, **93** (4), 246–51.

Mental Health Foundation/Camelot Foundation (2006) *Truth Hurts: Report of the National Inquiry in Self-Harm in Young People*, Mental Health Foundation/Camelot Foundation, London.

Metha, A. and McWhirter, E. (1997) Suicide ideation, depression, and stressful life events among gifted adolescents. *Journal of Education for the Gifted* **20**, 340–7.

Miller, L., Berg, J. and Archer, R. (1983) Openers: individuals who elicit intimate self-disclosure. *Journal of Personality and Social Psychology*, **44**, 1234–44.

Miller, S. (1980) Why having control reduces stress: if I can stop the roller coaster I don't want to get off, in *Human Helplessness: Theory and Applications* (eds J. Garber and M. Seligman), Academic Press, New York.

Molcho, A., Stanley, B. and Stanley, M. (1991) Biological studies and markers in suicide and attempted suicide. *International Clinical Psychopharmacology*, **6**, 77–92.

Moorley, S. (1995) Cognitive therapy, in *Individual Therapy* (ed. W. Dryden), Open University Press, Philadelphia.

Morano, C., Cisler, R. and Lemerond, J. (1993) Risk factors for adolescent suicidal behavior: loss, insufficient familial support, and hopelessness. *Adolescence*, **28** (112), 851–65.

Morgan, H. and Stanton, R. (1997) Suicide among psychiatric in-patients in a changing clinical scene. Suicidal ideation as a paramount index of short-term risk. *British Journal of Psychiatry*, **171**, 561–3.

Morgan, H., Burns-Cox, C., Pocock, H. *et al.* (1975) Deliberate self-harm: clinical and socio-economic characteristics of 368 patients. *British Journal of Psychiatry*, **127**, 564–74.

Morgan, H., Evans, M., Johnson, C. and Stanton, R. (1996) Can a lecture influence attitudes to suicide prevention? *Journal of the Royal Society of Medicine*, **89** (2), 87–90.

Morrison, L. and L'Heureux, J. (2001) Suicide and gay/lesbian/bisexual youth: implications for clinicians. *Journal of Adolescence*, **24**, 39–49.

Morrison, P. (1990) An example of the use of repertory grid technique in assessing nurses' self-perceptions of caring. *Nurse Education Today*, **10**, 253–9.

Muck-Seler, D., Jakovljevic, M. and Pivac, N. (1996) Platelet 5-HT concentrations and suicidal behaviour in recurrent major depression. *Journal of Affective Disorders*, **39** (1), 73–80.

Muehlenkamp, J. and Gutierrez, P. (2004) An investigation of differences between self-injurious behaviour and suicide attempts in a sample of adolescents. *Suicide and Life-Threatening Behavior*, **34** (1), 12–23.

Muller, A. and Poggenpoel, M. (1996) Patients' internal world experience of interacting with psychiatric nurses. *Archives of Psychiatric Nursing*, **10** (3), 143–50.

Murphy, G., McAleer, J. and O'Connor, F. (1984) Drug overdoses: a three year study at Altnagelvin Hospital, Londonderry. *Ulster Medical Journal*, **53**, 131–9.

Murphy, R. (2006) Mirror your life. *Daily Mirror*, 13 May 2006, p. 5.

Murray, W.H. (1947) *Mountaineering in Scotland*, J M Dent & Sons Ltd., London.

National Institute for Clinical Excellence (2004a) *Self-Harm: Short Term Physical and Psychological Management and Secondary Prevention of Self-Harm in Primary and Secondary Care*, NICE, London.

National Institute for Clinical Excellence (2004b) *Clinical Guideline 23. Depression: Management of Depression in Primary and Secondary Care*, NICE, London.

National Institute for Mental Health in England (NIMHE) (2003) *Personality Disorder: No Longer a Diagnosis of Exclusion*, NIMHE, London.

National Suicide Research Foundation (2002) *National Parasuicide Registry Ireland: Annual Report 2002*, National Suicide Research Foundation, Cork.

Neilson, P. and Brennan, W. (2001) The use of special observations: an audit within a psychiatric unit. *Journal of Psychiatric and Mental Health Nursing*, **8**, 147–55.

Nievaard, A. (1987) Communication climate and patient care: causes and effects of nurses' attitudes to patients. *Social Science and Medicine*, **24** (9), 77–784.

Noll, J., Horowitz, L., Bonanno, G. *et al.* (2003) Revictimization and self-harm in females who experienced childhood sexual abuse. *Journal of Interpersonal Violence*, **18** (12), 1452–147.

Nordentoft, M. and Rubin, P. (1993) Mental illness and social integration among suicide attempters in Copenhagen: comparison with the general population and a four-year follow-up-study of 100 patients. *Acta Psychiatrica Scandinavica*, **88** (4), 278–85.

Nordstrom, P., Ashberg, M., Abergwistedt, A. *et al.* (1995) Attempted suicide predicts risk in mood disorders. *Acta Psychiatrica Scandinavica*, **92** (5), 345–50.

Nordstrom, P., Samuelsson, M., Ashberg, M. *et al.* (1994) CSF 5-HIAA predicts suicide risk after attempted suicide. *Suicide and Life-Threatening Behavior*, **24** (1), 1–9.

O'Brien, S. and Stoll, K. (1977) Attitudes of medical and nursing staff towards self-poisoning patients in a London hospital. *International Journal of Nursing Studies*, **14**, 29–35.

Obrist, P. (1981) *Cardiovascular Psychophysiology: A Perspective*, Plenum, New York.

O'Carroll, P., Berman, A., Maris, R. *et al.* (1996) Beyond the Tower of Babel: a nomenclature for suicidology. *Suicide and Life-Threatening Behavior*, **26** (3), 237–52.

Oddy, J. (2006) *Daily Mirror*, 18 March 2006, p. 31.

Ohberg, A., Vuori, E., Ojanpera, I. *et al.* (1996) Alcohol and drugs in suicides. *British Journal of Psychiatry*, **169** (1), 75–80.

Osborne, M. (1989) Suicide and the response of the critical care nurse. *Holistic Nursing Practice*, **4** (1), 18–23.

O'Sullivan, M. and Ftizgerald, M. (1998) Suicidal ideation and acts of self-harm among Dublin school children. *Journal of Adolescence*, **21**, 427–33.

Owen, K. and Watson, N. (1995) Unemployment and mental health. *Journal of Psychiatric and Mental Health Nursing,* **2** (2), 63–71.

Owens, D., Dennis, M., Read, S. and Davis, N. (1994) Outcome of deliberate self-poisoning: an examination of risk factors for repetition. *British Journal of Psychiatry,* **165** (6), 797–801.

Owens, D., Horrocks, J. and House, A. (2002) Fatal and non-fatal repetition of self-harm. Systematic review. *British Journal of Psychiatry,* **181**, 193–9.

Pallikkathayil, L. and Morgan, S. (1988) Emergency department nurses' encounters with suicide attempters: a qualitative investigation. *Scholarly Inquiry for Nursing Practice,* **2** (3), 237–53.

Pan, P. and Lieh-Mak, F. (1989) A comparison between male and female parasuicides in Hong Kong. *Social Psychiatry and Psychiatric Epidemiology,* **24** (5), 253–7.

Panorama (2005) Bullying in schools. *British Broadcasting Corporation.* BBC1: 9 p.m. Sunday 10 April 2005.

Patel, A. (1975) Attitudes towards self-poisoning. *British Medical Journal,* **2** (5968), 426–9.

Paul, T., Schroeter, K., Dahme, B. *et al.* (2002) Self-injurious behavior in women with eating disorders. *American Journal of Psychiatry,* **159**, 408–11.

Paykel, E., Prusoff, B. and Myers, J. (1975) Suicide attempts and recent life events: a controlled comparison. *Archives of General Psychiatry,* **32**, 327–33.

Pembroke, L. (1998a) Self harm: a personal story (Part 1). *Mental Health Practice,* **2** (2), 20–4.

Pembroke, L. (1998b) Self harm: a personal story (Part 2). *Mental Health Practice,* **2** (3), 22–4.

Pembroke, L. (1998c) Only scratching the surface . . . self-harm. *Nursing Times,* **94** (27), 38–9.

Pembroke, L. and Smith, A. (1998) *Minimising the Damage from Self-Harm: The Guide for Friends, Relatives and Advocates Going with a Person who Self-Harms to an Accident and Emergency Department.* National Self-Harm Network, London.

Pennington, D. (1986) *Essential Social Psychology,* Edward Arnold, London.

Peplau, H. (1952) *Interpersonal Relations in Nursing: A Conceptual Frame of Reference for Psychodynamic Nursing,* Putnam, New York.

Peplau, H. (1994) Psychiatric mental health nursing: challenge and change. *Journal of Psychiatric and Mental Health Nursing,* **1** (1), 3–7.

Pierce, D. (1977) Suicidal intent in self-injury. *British Journal of Psychiatry,* **130**, 377–85.

Pillay, A. (1987) Factors precipitating parasuicide among young South African Indians. *Psychological Reports,* **61** (2), 545–6.

Pillay, A. and Vawda, N. (1989) Alcohol related parasuicides among married people. *South African Medical Journal,* **75** (3), 120–1.

Pinto, A., Whisman, A. and Conwell, Y. (1998) Reasons for living in a clinical sample of adolescents. *Journal of Clinical Adolescence,* **21** (4), 397–405.

Pirkola, S., Sohlman, B. and Wahlbeck, K. (2005) The characteristics of suicides within a week of discharge after psychiatric hospitalisation – a nationwide register study. http://www.biomedcentral.com/1471-244X/5/32 (September 2006).

Platt, S. and Kreitman, N. (1990) Long term trends in parasuicide and unemployment in Edinburgh, 1968–1987. *Social Psychiatry and Psychiatric Epidemiology*, **25**, 56–61.

Platt, S. and Salter, D. (1987) A comparative investigation of health workers' attitudes towards parasuicide. *Social Psychiatry*, **22** (4), 202–8.

Platt, S., Hawton, K., Kreitman, N. *et al.* (1988) Recent clinical and epidemiological trends in parasuicide in Edinburgh and Oxford: a tale of two cities. *Psychological Medicine*, **18** (2), 405–18.

Pokorny, A. (1974) A scheme for classifying suicidal behaviors, in *The Prediction of Suicide* (eds A. Beck, H. Resnick and D. Lettieri), The Charles Press, Philadelphia, PA.

van Praag, H. (1983) CSF 5-HIAA and suicide in non-depressed schizophrenics. *Lancet*, **ii**, 977–8.

van Praag, H. (2001) About the biological interface between psychotraumatic experiences and affective dysregulation, in *Understanding Suicidal Behaviour: The Suicidal Process, Approach to Research, Treatment and Prevention* (ed. K. Van Heeringen), John Wiley & Sons, Inc., New York.

van Praag, H., Korf, J. and Puite, J. (1970) 5-Hydroxindoleacetic acid levels in the cerebrospinal fluid of depressive patients treated with probenecid. *Nature*, **225**, 1259–60.

Pritchard, C. (1992) Is there a link between suicide in young men and unemployment? A comparison of the U.K. with other European Community Countries. *British Journal of Psychiatry*, **160**, 750–6.

Pritchard, C. (1995) Unemployment, age, gender and regional suicide in England and Wales 1974–1990: a harbinger of increased suicide for the 1990s. *British Journal of Social Work*, **25** (6), 767–90.

Ramon, S., Bancroft, J. and Skrimshire, A. (1975) Attitudes towards self-poisoning among physicians and nurses in a general hospital. *British Journal of Psychiatry*, **127**, 257–64.

Ran, M.-S., Wu, Q.-H., Conwell, Y. *et al.* (2004) Suicidal behaviour among inpatients with schizophrenia and mood disorders in Chengdu, China. *Suicide and Life-Threatening Behavior*, **34** (3), 311–19.

Rankin, W. (1989) Teenage suicide. *Journal of Pediatric Nursing*, **4**, 130–1.

Ray, S. (1996) Rights and responsibilities: suicide and the decision to die. *Mental Health Nursing*, **16** (3), 7.

Redfield-Jamison, K. (1995) *The Unquiet Mind: A Memoir of Moods and Madness*, Picador, London.

Reinherz, H., Giaconia, R., Silverman, M. *et al.* (1995) Early psychosocial risk for adolescent suicidal ideation and attempts. *Journal of the American Academy of Child and Adolescent Psychiatry*, **34**, 599–611.

Remafedi, G., Farrow, J. and Deisher, R. (1991) Risk factors for attempted suicide in gay and bisexual youth. *Pediatrics*, **87** (6), 869–75.

Rigby, K. (2000) Effects of peer victimization in schools and perceived social support on adolescent well-being. *Journal of Adolescence*, **23**, 57–68.

Riggs, S., Alariom, A. and McHorneym, C. (1990) Health risk behaviors and attempted suicide in adolescents who report prior maltreatment. *Journal of Pediatrics*, **116** (5), 815–21.

Rihmer, Z. (1996) Strategies of suicide prevention: focus on health care. *Journal of Affective Disorders*, **39** (2), 83–91.

Rivers, I. (1997) Respecting differences in a changing society – Lesbian, Gay, and Bisexual Voices. Paper delivered to a conference in St Columb's Park House, Derry, Northern Ireland on the 15 February 1997.

Rogers, C. (1951) *Client-Centred Therapy*, Houghton Mifflin, Boston.

Rogers, C. (1961) *On Becoming a Person*, Houghton Mifflin, Boston.

Rogers, C. (1975) Empathetic: an unappreciated way of being. *The Counselling Psychologist*, **5**, 2–10.

Romans, S., Martin, J. and Anderson, J. (1995) Sexual abuse in childhood and deliberate self-harm. *American Journal of Psychiatry*, **152**, 1336–42.

Ross, C. and Mirowsky, J. (1995) Does unemployment affect health? *Journal of Health and Social Behavior*, **36** (2), 230–43.

Rowly, J., Ganter, K. and Fitzpatrick, C. (2001) Suicidal thoughts and acts in Irish adolescents. *Irish Journal of Psychological Medicine*, **18** (3), 82–6.

Roy, A. (1996) Aetiology of secondary depression in male alcoholics. *British Journal of Psychiatry*, **169** (6), 753–7.

Roy, A., DeJong, J. and Linnoila, M. (1989) Cerebrospinal fluid monoamine metabolites and suicidal behaviour in depressed patients. *Archives of General Psychiatry*, **46**, 609–12.

Roy, A., Mazonson, A. and Pickar, D. (1984) Attempted suicide in schizophrenia. *British Journal of Psychiatry*, **144**, 303–6.

Royal College of Psychiatrists (1996) *Report of the Confidential Inquiry into Homicides and Suicides by Mentally Ill People*, Royal College of Psychiatrists, London.

Rudd, M. (1997) What's in a name. . . . *Suicide and Life-Threatening Behavior*, **27** (3), 326–7.

Rudd, M., Joiner, T. and Rajab, M. (2001) *Treating Suicidal Behaviour: An Effective, Time-Limited Approach*, The Guilford Press, New York.

Runeson, B. (2002) Suicide after parasuicide. *British Medical Journal*, **325**, 1125–6.

Russell, T. and Morrill, C. (1989) Adding a systematic touch to rationale-emotive therapy for families. *Journal of Mental Health Counseling*, **11**, 184–92.

Rygnestad, T. (1988) A prospective 5-year follow-up study of self-poisoned patients. *Acta Psychiatrica Scandinavica*, **77**, 328–31.

Sainsbury Centre for Mental Health (1998) *Acute Problems: A Survey of the Quality of Care in Acute Psychiatric Wards*, The Sainsbury Centre for Mental Health, London.

Sainsbury Centre for Mental Health (2002) *Acute Inpatient Care*, The Sainsbury Centre for Mental Health, London.

Sainsbury Centre for Mental Health (2006) *We Need to Talk: The Case for Psychological Therapies on the NHS*, The Sainsbury Centre for Mental Health, London.

Sakinofsky, I., Roberts, R., Brown, Y. *et al.* (1990) Problem resolution and repetition of parasuicide: a prospective study. *British Journal of Psychiatry*, **156**, 395–9.

Samaritans (2006) http://www.samaritans.org.uk/know/information/suicide_stats. shtm (21 December 2006).

Samuelsson, M., Wiklander, M., Asberg, M. and Saveman, B. (2000) Psychiatric care as seen by the attempted suicide patient. *Journal of Advanced Nursing*, **32** (3), 635–43.

van der Sande, R., Buskens, E., Van Der Graff, Y. and Van Engeland, H. (1997) Psychosocial intervention following suicide attempt: a systematic review of treatment interventions. *Acta Psychiatrica Scandinavica*, **96** (1), 43–50.

Schmidt, E., O'Neal, P. and Robins, E. (1954) Evaluation of suicide attempts as a guide to therapy. *Journal of the American Medical Association*, **155**, 549–57.

Schmidtke, A., Bille-Brahe, U., Deleo, D. *et al.* (1996) Attempted suicide in Europe: rates, trends, and sociodemographic characteristics of suicide attempters during the period 1989–1992 – results of the WHO/Euro Multicenter Study on Parasuicide. *Acta Psychiatrica Scandinavica*, **93** (5), 327–38.

Seligman, M. (1975) *Helplessness*, Freeman, San Francisco.

Selye, H. (1956) *The Stress of Life*, McGraw-Hill, New York.

Seymour, L. and Groove, B. (2005) *Workplace Interventions for People with Common Mental Health Problems*, British Occupational Health Research Foundation, London.

Shaffer, D., Garland, A., Gould, M. *et al.* (1988) Preventing teenage suicide: a critical review. *Journal of the American Academy of Child and Adolescent Psychiatry*, **27**, 675–87.

Shea, S.C. (2002) *The Practical Art of Suicide Assesment: A Guide for Mental Health Professionals and Substance Abuse Counselors*, John Wiley & Sons, Inc., New Jersey.

Sheldon, B. (1995) *Cognitive-Behavioural Therapy*, Routledge, New York.

Shneidman, E. (1993) *Suicide as Psychache: A Clinical Approach to Self-Destructive Behavior*, Jason Aronson, Northvale, NJ.

Shneidman, E. (1968) Classification of suicidal phenomena. *Bulletin of Suicidology*, **2**, 1–9.

Shneidman, E. (1985) *Definition of Suicide*, John Wiley & Sons, Inc., New York.

Shneidman, E. (1992) What do suicides have in common? Summary of the psychological approach, in *Suicide: Guidelines for Assessment, Management and Treatment* (ed. B. Bongar), Oxford University Press, Oxford, pp. 3–15.

Shneidman, E. (2005) Prediction of suicide revisited: a brief methodological note. *Suicide and Life-Threatening Behavior*, **35** (1), 1–2.

Sidley, G. and Renton, J. (1996) General nurses' attitudes to patients who self-harm. *Nursing Standard*, **10** (30), 32–6.

Silove, D., George, G. and Bhavani-Sankaram, V. (1987) Parasuicide: interaction between inadequate parenting and recent interpersonal stress. *Australian and New Zealand Journal of Psychiatry*, **21** (2), 221–8.

Silver, M., Bohnert, M., Beck, A. *et al.* (1971) Relation of depression of attempted suicide and seriousness of intent. *Archives of General Psychiatry*, **25**, 573–6.

Silverman, M. (2005) What's in a name: The language of Suicidology. Suicide Prevention Resource Centre. Discussion Series November 2005.

Silverman, M. (2006) The language of suicidology. *Suicide and Life-Threatening Behaviour*, **36** (5), 519–32.

Skegg, K., Nada-Raja, S. and Dickson, N. (2003) Sexual orientation and self-harm in men and women. *American Journal of Psychiatry*, **160**, 541–6.

Smith, M. (1998) *Working With Self Harm: Victim to Victor*, Handsell Publishing, Birmingham.

Smith, S. (2002) Perceptions of service provision for clients who self-injure in the absence of expressed suicidal intent. *Journal of Psychiatric and Mental Health Nursing*, **9**, 595–601.

Snow, L. (2002) Prisoners' motives for self-injury and attempted suicide. *British Journal of Forensic Practice*, **4** (4), 18–29.

Snow, L., Paton, J., Oram, C. and Teers, R. (2002) Self-inflicted deaths during 2001: an analysis of trends. *British Journal of Forensic Practice*, **4** (4), 3–17.

Sorenson, S. and Rutter, C. (1991) Transgenerational patterns of suicide attempt. *Journal of Consulting and Clinical Psychology*, **59**, 861–6.

Speck, R. (1967) Psychotherapy of the social network of a schizophrenic family. *Family Processes*, **6**, 208–14.

Speijer, N. and Diekstra, R. (1980) *Assisted Suicide: A Study of the Problems Related to Self-Chosen Death*, van Loghun Slaterur, Peventer.

Stack, S. and Wasserman, I. (1995) Marital status, alcohol abuse, and attempted suicide: a logit model. *Journal of Addictive Studies*, **14** (2), 43–51.

Stark, C., Smith, H. and Hall, D. (1994) Increase in parasuicide in Scotland. *British Medical Journal*, **308**, 1569–70.

Stenager, E. and Jensen, K. (1994) Attempted suicide and contact with primary health authorities. *Acta Psychiatrica Scandinavica*, **90** (2), 109–13.

Stravynski, A. and Boyer, R. (2001) Loneliness in relation to suicide ideation and parasuicide: a population-wide study. *Suicide and Life-Threatening Behavior*, **31** (1), 32–40.

Suarez-Almazor, M., Newman, C., Hanson, J. and Bruera, E. (2002) Attitudes of terminally ill cancer patients about euthanasia and assisted suicide: predominance of psychosocial determinants and beliefs over symptom distress and subsequent survival. *Journal of Clinical Oncology*, **20** (8), 2134–41.

Sykes, J. (ed.) (1987) *The Concise Oxford Dictionary*, 7th edn, Oxford University Press, New York.

Thoits, P. (1994) Stressors and problem-solving: the individual as a psychological activist. *Journal of Health and Social Behavior*, **35** (2), 143–60.

Toch, H. (1975) *Men in Crisis*, Aldine, Chicago.

Trower, P., Casey, A. and Dryden, W. (1989) *Cognitive-Behavioural Counselling in Action*, Sage Publications, London.

Truax, C. and Mitchell, K. (1971) Research on certain therapist interpersonal skills in relation to process and outcome, in *Handbook of Psychotherapy and Behavioural Change* (eds A. Bergin and S. Garfield), John Wiley & Sons, Inc., New York.

Turano, R. (1996) Follow the leader. *Emergency Medical Services*, **25** (5), 43–4.61.

Turner, R. (1982) Parasuicide in an urban general practice, 1970–1979. *Journal of the Royal College of General Practitioners*, **32**, 273–81.

Turner, R. and Marino, F. (1994) Social support and social structure: a descriptive epidemiology. *Journal of Health and Social Behavior*, **35** (3), 193–212.

Tyrer, P. (2000) *Personality Disorders: Diagnosis, Management and Course*, 2nd edn, Butterworth Heinemann, Oxford.

Vassilas, C. and Morgan, H. (1993) General practitioners' contact with victims of suicide. *British Medical Journal*, **307** (6899), 300–1.

Verkes, R., Kerkhof, G., Hengeveld, G. *et al.* (1996) Suicidality, circadian activity rhythms and platelet serotonergic measures in patients with recurrent suicidal behaviour. *Acta Psychiatrica Scandinavica*, **93** (1), 27–34.

Vivekananda, K. (2000) Integrating models for understanding self-injury. *Psychotherapy in Australia*, **7**, 18–25.

Wagner, B., Wong, S. and Jobes, D. (2002) Mental health professionals' determinations of adolescent suicide attempts. *Suicide and Life-Threatening Behaviour*, **32** (3), 284–300.

Warman, D., Forman, E., Henriques, G. *et al.* (2004) Suicidality and psychosis: beyond depression and hopelessness. *Suicide and Life-Threatening Behavior*, **34** (1), 77–86.

Waterhouse, J. and Platt, S. (1990) General hospital admission in the management of parasuicide: a randomised controlled trial. *British Journal of Psychiatry*, **156**, 236–42.

Watson, J. and McDougall, W. (1929) *The Battle of Behaviorism*, Norton, New York.

Watson, J.C. (2002) Re-visioning empathy, in *Humanistic Psychotherapies; Handbook of Research and Practice* (eds D.J. Cain and J. Seeman), American Psychological association, Washington, DC, pp. 445–71.

Weaver, T., Chard, K., Mechanic, M. *et al.* (2004) Self-injurious behaviors, PTSD arousal, and general health complaints within a treatment-seeking sample of sexually abused women. *Journal of Interpersonal Violence*, **19** (5), 558–75.

Westermeyer, J. and Harrow, M. (1989) Early phases of schizophrenia and depression: prediction of suicide, in *Depression in Schizophrenics* (eds R. Williams and J. Dalby), Plenum, New York, pp. 153–69.

Western Investment for Health (2006) Mental health in unemployed men. http://www.westernifh.org (October 2006).

Whittington, D. and McLaughlin, C. (2000) Finding time for patients: an exploration of nurses' time allocation in an acute psychiatric setting. *Journal of Psychiatric and Mental Health Nursing*, **7**, 259–68.

Wilkinson, D. (1989) *Depression: Recognition and Treatment in General Practice*, Radcliffe Medical Press, Oxford.

Wilkinson, G. and Bacon, N. (1984) A clinical and epidemiological survey of parasuicides and suicide in Edinburgh schizophrenics. *Psychological Medicine*, **14** (4), 899–912.

Wilson, K., Stelzer, J., Bergman, J. *et al.* (1995) Problem solving, stress, and coping in adolescent suicide attempts. *Suicide and Life-Threatening Behavior*, **25**, 241–52.

Wolf, Z. (1986) The caring concept and nurse identified caring behaviours. *Topics in Clinical Nursing*, **8**, 84–93.

Woods, M. (1990) Counselling services for adolescents. *Nursing Standard*, **4** (21), 17–19.

World Health Organization (1985) *Targets for Health for All: Targets in Support of the European Regional Strategy for Health for All*, WHO, Copenhagen.

World Health Organization (1992) *The ICD-10 Classification of Mental and Behavioural Disorders: Clinical Descriptions and Diagnostic Guidelines*, WHO, Geneva.

World Health Organization (2001) *Mental Health, New Understanding, New Hope*, WHO, Geneva.

World Health Organization (2002a) *World Report on Violence and Health*, WHO, Geneva.

World Health Organization (2002b) *Prevention and Promotion in Mental Health: Evidence and Research*, World Health Organization, Geneva.

Yarden, P. (1974) Observations on suicide in chronic schizophrenics. *Comprehensive Psychiatry*, **15**, 325–33.

Zahl, D. and Hawton, K. (2004) Repetition of deliberate self-harm and subsequent suicide risk: long term follow-up study of 11 583 patients. *British Journal of Psychiatry*, **185**, 70–5.

Zest (2006) Healing the Hurt. Conference in the City Hotel. Derry, Northern Ireland. February 2006.

Zest (2003) Healing the Hurt. Conference in the City Hotel, Derry, Northern Ireland. October 2003.

Index